in-Training
2020 In Our Words

ALSO BY PAGER PUBLICATIONS, INC.

—

in-Training: Stories from Tomorrow's Physicians

Family Doc Diary: A Resident Physician's Reflections in Fifty-Two Entries

in-Training: Stories from Tomorrow's Physicians, Volume 2

Salve: Words For The Journey

The Doctor Will Be Late

in-Training
2020 In Our Words

Peer-edited narratives written by medical students about their experiences throughout the year 2020

edited by
Pallavi Juneja & Samuel Rouleau

PAGER PUBLICATIONS, INC.
a 501c3 non-profit literary corporation

in-Training: 2020 In Our Words

Copyright © 2021 by Pager Publications, Inc.. All rights reserved.

Published by Pager Publications, Inc. at pagerpublications.org.

Printed in the United States of America.

No part of this book may be used or reproduced in any manner whatsoever without written permission from Pager Publications, Inc., except in the case of brief quotations with proper reference embodied in critical articles and reviews.

All patient names, protected health information, and any other identifying information in this book have been changed to protect patient privacy.

Cover art by Shivani Ghoshal.
Book design by Ajay Major.

First Printing: 2021

ISBN-13: 978-0-578-96784-4

2020

by Samuel Rouleau

Our dreams strewn across barren land —
fractured communities, little love, who are we?

We dissolve into bitterness, this virus feasts —
its appetite leaves despair.

(Only a biological phenomenon, yet I take it personally)

Some days, I only feel disillusion of the soul
that yearns for bear hugs, game nights, Nana's pecan pie.

Masked cheeks give away strangers' smiles.
Here we are, looking for ripe avocados, together.

Silent gratitude for a moment shared.
We feel this ache, this suffering.

We are each other.

Contents

in-Training and Pager Publications, Inc. Mission Statements	x
in-Training Editorial Board	xi
Acknowledgements	xii
Preface by Pallavi Juneja & Samuel Rouleau	xiii

The Pandemic • preclinical — 1

Rising Out of the Ruin by Trisha Kaundinya	3
Starting from Scratch: Building M1 Teamwork During the Pandemic by Jen Geller	6
From the Window by Thomas Amburn	9
Step 1 in the Time of COVID by Paavani Reddy and Apshara Ravichandran	11
Silver Lining by Samantha M. Rodriguez	15
Lessons from Quarantine by Sylvia Guerra	17

The Pandemic • clinical — 20

Should Medical Students Continue Clinical Rotations During COVID-19? by Canon Brodar	21
Medical Ethics in the Time of COVID-19: A Call for Critical Reflection by Adrian Anzaldua	24
The Role of Third-Year Medical Students During the Pandemic by Matthew Henry	29
Frontline by Maria Hanna	33

The Pandemic • socio-legal — 35

COVID-19 Lockdowns: Are They Legal? by Meghan Sharma	36
Precedented: Historical Guidance on Freedom and Health in COVID-19 by Adrian Anzaldua	40
Cruel and Unusual Punishment: Incarceration in a Pandemic by Olivia Rizzo and Brianna Sohl	44
496 Beds: Medical Students Call to Action by Hannah Roach, Kristin Speigel, Jenny Nguyen, Emma Schanzenbach, & Natalie Marie Dicenzo	47

51   Intimate Reflections • inward

- 52   A Nation On My Shoulders by Neha Deo
- 53   Lessons on Coronavirus From My Great Grandpa Saul by Samantha Greissman
- 56   three machines by Kirsten Myers
- 58   CLL (Child Learning Love) by Gabriel Davis
- 60   Pattern Recognition by Samantha Schroth
- 62   My First Stitch: A Dramatic Retelling by Eric Bethea

65   Intimate Reflections • outward

- 66   Buddy by John Carlo Pasco
- 69   Restrained by Madeline Fryer
- 72   Grief Unanswered by Sharon Hsu
- 74   "I Can't Be Here Anymore" by Vidiya Sathananthan
- 77   Emptied by Rma Kumra
- 79   The Infinite by Meagan Campbell

81   Reimagining #MedEd • culture

- 82   Yes, Doctor by Rohan Patel
- 85   Welcome to Medicine by Apshara Ravichandran
- 88   The Vulnerability of Our Patients and Ourselves by Rachel Fields
- 91   Becoming More Emotionally Intelligent, Adaptive Physician-Leaders by Ashten Duncan

94   Reimagining #MedEd • wellness

- 95   Medical Students Do Not Owe You Their Trauma by Tabitha Moses
- 98   Do I Belong Here? by Rohan Patel
- 100   A Defense of My Suicidal Peers by May Chammaa
- 103   Soulful Medicine by Eric Bethea

Reimagining #MedEd • progress — 107

Life as Chimera: When Life Combines With Itself by George E. Tsourdinis — 108
Well, It Happened: Step 1 Will Become Pass/Fail — 111
by Pranav Reddy, MD, MPA, Kunal K. Sindhu, MD, and Bryan Carmody, MD, MPH
Unpacking the "Insult" of Being Called a Nurse as a Female Physician — 114
by Jessa Fogel
More Than Skin Deep: Underrepresentation of Brown and Black Skin — 116
by Maiya Smith and Tyler Thorne
You're Not a Bold, Knowledgeable Medical Student — You're Just White — 119
by Nat Mulkey

Advocacy: This Is Our Lane • racism — 123

The Autopsy Report of Mr. George Floyd by Amal Cheema — 124
Images of Violence Unravel Us — And Our Communities by Anna Ayala — 126
This is Water: A Perspective on Race from a White Male — 128
by Caleb Sokolowski
Physicians' Role in Addressing Racism by Swetha Tummala — 130
A Few Words on Health Disparity in the Asian American Community — 133
by Jasmine Lam
It's A Lot by Holly Ingram — 135

Advocacy: This Is Our Lane • refugees — 138

Providers, Not Puppets by Yasmine Suliman — 139
Forced Hysterectomies in ICE Detention Centers — 142
by Lucy Brown, Meghana Kudrimoti, Minji Kim and Candise Johnson
The Largest Humanitarian Catastrophe of Yemen by Leah Sarah Peer — 144
Aylan by Sharon Hsu — 147

Advocacy: This Is Our Lane • public health — 148

Doctors for Democracy by Rob Palmer — 149
We Have a Cost Crisis in Medicine by Caleb Sokolowski — 151
Medical Students Call to Flatten the Curve on Climate Change — 154
by Sarah Hsu, Natasha Sood, Harleen Marwah, Ellen Townley and Sarah Schear

References — 158

in-Training Mission Statement

in-Training is the online peer-reviewed publication for medical students,
founded in April 2012 by Ajay Major and Aleena Paul,
medical students at Albany Medical College.

in-Training is the agora of the medical student community,
the collaborative center for discourse and
the free expression of our voices.

in-Training seeks to:

promote students' self-reflection that is both authentic and empowering;

cultivate a diverse, inclusive and interconnected community;

and shape the medical student experience, and in doing so,
the future of medicine.

Pager Publications, Inc. Mission Statement

Pager Publications, Inc. is a 501c3 nonprofit literary organization
that curates and supports peer-edited publications
for the medical education community.

The organization strives to provide students and educators
with dedicated spaces for the free expression of their distinctive voices.

Pager Publications, Inc. was officially incorporated in January 2015
by its founders Ajay Major, Aleena Paul and Erica Fugger
to provide administrative and financial support for
in-Training and other publications.

in-Training
the agora of the medical student community

Pallavi Juneja & Sam Rouleau
Editors-in-Chief

Ajay Major & Aleena Paul
Founders and Editors-in-Chief Emeriti

Brian James & Alina Siddiqui
Managing Editors

Vikas Bhatt & Joseph Ladowski
Ria Pal & Andrew Kadlec
Amelia Mackarey & Nihaal Mehta
Emma Martin & James Lee
Editors-in-Chief Emeriti

Editors

Zofia Hetman	Aida Haddad	Alex Carter
Steven Duncan	Jennifer Li	Michael Spears
Coco Thomas	Julie Yi	Holly Ingram
Gabe Davis	Buckley McCall	Lily Foley
Max Chou	Valerie Chuy	Ashten Duncan
	Farhan Salman	
	Bhargavi Dhanireddy	

Editors Emeriti

Lydia Boyette	Will Jaffee	Tim Beck	Allison Lyle
Denise Mai	Matthew Lenardis	Jacob Kammerman	Steven Lange
Olivia Abbate	Luke Fraley	Brenna Brown	Nita Chen
Kshama Bhyravabhotla	Romela Petrosyan	Jessica Downing	Nisha Hariharan
Yuli Zhu	Evan Torline	Steph Cockrill	Tolulope Omojokun
Ileana Horattas	Roshini Selladurai	Hormuz Nicolwala	Dustin Nowotny
Brent Schnipke	Lisa Tran	Sanjay Salgado	Lexy Adam
Angelica D'Aiello	Daniel Coleman	Jimmy Tam Huy Pham	Lytani Wilson
Phyllis Ying	David Yu	Kimberly Ku	Melanie Watt
Samantha Margulies	Heba Albasha	Sasha Yakhkind	Abishag Suresh
Nina Nguyen	Sandy Tadros	Laura Mucenski	Visvarath Varadarajan
Lindsey McDaniel	Elaine Hsiang	Francis Dailey	Lauren Bojarski
Claire Drom	Jasmine Gite	Dragos Rezeanu	Clara Thomson
Anne Nzuki	Jennifer Li	Nikki Nametz	Joseph Gottwald
Chris Deans	Anna Qian	Emily Lu	Amira Athanasios
Diane Brackett	Sohini Khan	Brent Bjornsen	Pompeyo Quesada
Natalie Wilcox	Meena Darden	Theresa Yang	Slavena Salve Nissan
Chelcie Soroka	Jane Liao	Amol Utrankar	Sarah Garvey
Kate Joyce	Nisitha Sengottuvel	Mansi Sheth	Jason Bunn
Jarna Shah	Elizabeth Shay	Eric Donahue	Pardis Pooshpas

Acknowledgements

Our gratitude extends to all the contributors to *in-Training*.
Your vulnerability and reflections spark insight
into our own journeys to physicianhood.

Thank you to the *in-Training* editorial staff,
who tirelessly shaped the content of this publication.

To Dr. Ajay Major and Dr. Aleena Paul,
this book would have remained only an idea
without your steadfast support and direction.

We are deeply grateful for the cover work by Dr. Shivani Ghoshal
and the chapter artwork by Dr. Maryam Khalil.

Preface

by Pallavi Juneja and Samuel Rouleau
Editors of *in-Training: 2020 In Our Words*

For those who undertake the journey to physicianhood, medical school is often an inherently unprecedented experience.

Among the unique challenges that we face are working long hours, learning high volumes of information, and fitting in with the diverse medical team — all the while balancing our personal lives. The year of 2020 made all that even harder still.

The COVID-19 pandemic altered our training experience, with some students called up to the front lines and others sent home. The protests for racial justice made us question our responsibility to society — both as and beyond our roles as doctors-in-training. And in an election year, we educated ourselves and each other about issues of health care policy. Humanitarian crises around the world shook us, and the climate concerned us. Along the way, medical school fundamentally changed.

This book is meant to capture that force of change. As the editors-in-chief of *in-Training*, we are grateful for the privilege to share the voices of medical students. In training, we often feel that our voices soften or go silent altogether. Here, we aim to amplify the unique medical student experience of 2020. Poems, opinions, stories and statements — proudly, we share the subsequent work, created by more than 40 medical students from around the globe.

In the next 52 pieces, we tell our stories from the 52 weeks that comprised 2020 — in our words.

Yours-in-training,

Pallavi Juneja and Samuel Rouleau
Editors-in-Chief of *in-Training*
Class of 2021 at Wake Forest School of Medicine
and Class of 2021 at Mayo Clinic Alix School of Medicine

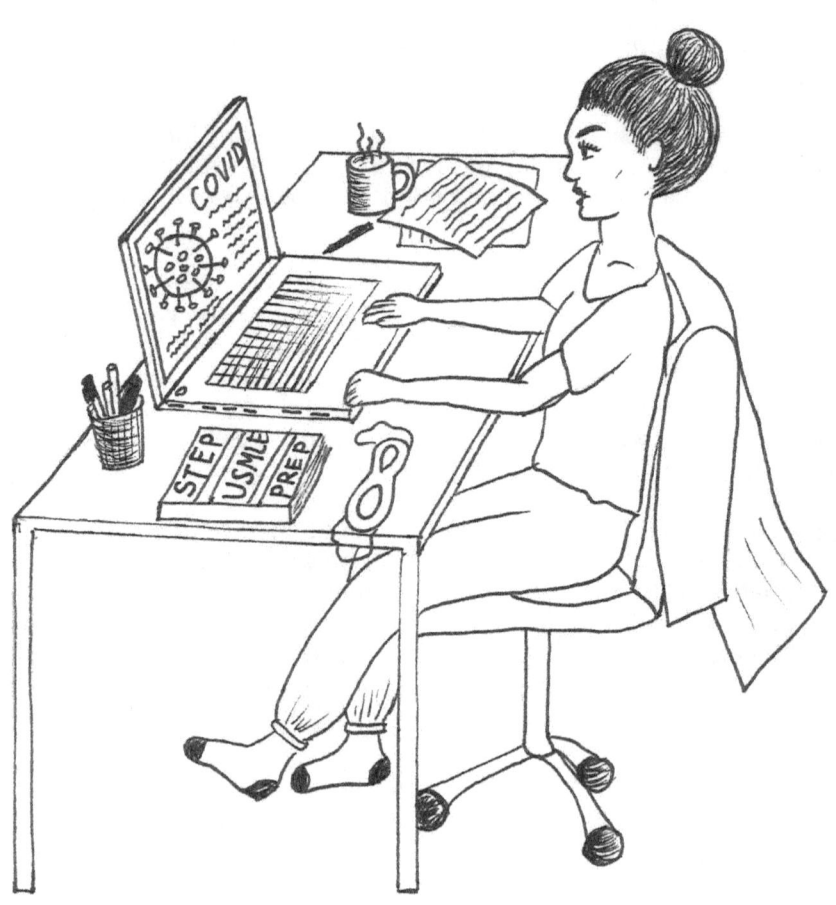

The Pandemic

•

preclinical

Rising Out of the Ruin
October 29, 2020

Trisha Kaundinya
Northwestern University Feinberg School of Medicine
Class of 2024

I wish it were different —
Dying patients, struggling hospitals, overworked health care workers,
topsy-turvy economies, politicized safety precautions, and the uncertainty
of tomorrow.

Rising caseloads,
or success with social distancing.
New guidelines from the CDC,
or permission to see family and friends in person.

The violent death of George Floyd, preceded by those of
Breonna Taylor,
Ahmaud Arbery,
Trayvon Martin,
Michael Brown,
thousands of others.

Opening our eyes, which have intentionally looked

                                                          the other way

since the age of slavery to police brutality.

Systemic racism: a driver of the damage and hurt that it has
uniquely caused our Black community.

And its penetration into the soul of our industries, health care systems,
of redlining, or the dramatic
disparities in maternal mortality.

A pandemic and tragic, racism-
induced deaths — causing us to redefine what normal should look like.

Both physical changes, like social distancing guidelines
and work-from-home orders,
and emotional ones such as mitigating the health care access gap
for Black populations.

What should our new communities prioritize? What should our health care systems do to create an equitable network?

—

Our medical school acceptance and enrollment —
such an exciting and special moment.
Learning about an online transition.

Should I take a gap year?

Clinics turned to Zoom demonstrations, orientation potlucks turned to microwave single-serve meals at home.

Not the same training as thousands of colleagues before us.
Will it be enough?

When will putting on that white coat lead to mentored patient encounters? Face-to-face conversations? In-person problem-solving?

Hoping for a routine, and yet
recognizing that returning to normal is not the outcome.

—

The process of bettering our health systems starts with us new trainees being actively anti-racist.
It starts with us educating ourselves on pandemic legislation
and the emergence of telehealth.

Recognizing the beaming opportunity and promise in this moment for us is difficult.

But it exists.

THE PANDEMIC

There are unique benefits to starting now:
Getting to train amidst a real-life case study of the value of medicine;
Seeing issues first-hand in our hospital networks
that we will now have the agency to change.

The gravity of this moment is taxing,
and the ambiguity is unsettling as a student.

We do not want to burden our mentors,
as their management of patients right now is the priority.

We just want to do this massive
academic,
personal,
professional,
financial
undertaking justice.

Justice will be to do right by our patients one day.

So,
whatever it takes —
the online start,
the social distancing,
the social justice training,
the privilege checks —
that's what we will do.

Entering medicine is an honor.
A pandemic will not undermine this honor.
Here we are! The next generation of medicine, rising out of the rubble.
Ready to learn and build a brighter medical system.

Starting from Scratch: Building M1 Teamwork During the Pandemic

November 4, 2020

Jen Geller
Rutgers Robert Wood Johnson Medical School
Class of 2024

MY FINGERS TRACED THE CRACK between each brick, feeling the uneven texture of granules and cement — something I have done when I am nervous since walking the hallways of elementary school. The July day was humid, and the sun beamed down with relentless heat and heavy humidity, making breathing a more conscious effort. Taking in as much breeze as we could and venturing to find shady places to stand, over 150 medical students collected — at a distance from one another with masks covering our faces — to commence our medical school journey as a new family.

None of us pictured beginning medical school in a pandemic. Most of us are still in shock we were admitted to medical school owing to severe imposter syndrome. Despite the exceedingly virtual nature of the fall semester — as of now, our only in-person activities are optional anatomy labs — we have hitherto made the most of this experience. Undeterred by the inability to partake in many in-person activities as a class, we are fostering meaningful relationships with our peers online and in person.

It is a well-known phenomenon that teamwork is absolutely crucial to being a physician who can provide the best quality of care to patients. When I applied to medical school in the first place, my pre-health advising office emphasized teamwork as one of the thirteen American Association of Medical Colleges (AAMC) core competencies of being a physician.[1]

Medicine is a team sport, and I do not just mean with other doctors. There is a network of hospital workers that ranges from doctors, nurses and physicians assistants to interpreters, dietitians and social workers, who all play a role in ensuring that our patients receive the best quality of care.[2] The mentality of working together towards a common goal is imperative far beyond the walls of medical school.

Everyone brings a different knowledge base to the table, and when we all come together, we create an entity even more powerful than a summation of our separate parts. According to the American College of Physicians (ACP), teamwork is one of the most essential parts of medical school, not only in the pre-clinical setting but also in clinical rotations and internship.[3] The ACP adds that it takes "humility, social skills and understanding to resolve conflict" between team members.

In the pre-clinical years, this is important in study groups when there are many different ways of learning the large amounts of material to be learned. Training to improve those skills at the pre-clinical level will make teamwork far less foreign later in training and throughout our career. Finding the right people to study with and to learn from will ultimately make everyone involved successful.

However, with the rise of COVD-19, finding the right teams for pre-clinical years is not as easy as when we could all simply meet for a meal after class or go to a student organization meeting.

Remember that humid July day? That was when my incoming medical school class recited the Hippocratic Oath and received white coats without families beside us. But we quickly realized that we did have something else: each other. Our new family that we started and continue to create day after day.

Orientation week was filled with socially distant get-togethers, ice-breaker games and quiet moments to get to know each other on a deeper level. Despite the fact that after orientation our formal in-person meetups became fewer and further between, we used our foundation to catapult ourselves into the stream of teamwork absolutely critical to driving our medical school success.

After finishing my first course in medical school, I can easily say that we really are in this together, and the importance of teamwork in medical education has only been magnified. It is hard to believe that I just met some of my peers in the past several months, for it feels significantly longer.

There is something to be said for persevering under an abnormal situation with a shared experience. We have turned walks in our housing development, journeys through nearby parks and study sessions with outdoor meal breaks into standard parts of our school lives. The bonds we form will remain in place long after our four years in medical school as we continue our friendships while pursuing careers in different specialties.

Admittedly, we did start ahead of the game by finding each other and building those support systems before school even began. One classmate, a very good friend of mine now, started hosting Zoom "happy hours" starting back in April, so we were virtually very familiar with each other. But there was something so different about orientation, seeing and waving to each other for the first time. We make jokes all the time now about how we are each taller or shorter than we thought after only meeting over Zoom for so long. We did not know who we would end up close with or who we would study the various porphyrias and trinucleotide-repeat disorders with for hours on end, but we did find each other and will continue to find what works best for us.

Like the beginning of any new step, the start of medical school was terrifying. The transition was made more difficult by not having the opportunity to sit in a lecture hall, take in the loads of information we need to learn, or eat lunch with each other before lab. However, with the capacity to connect safely, we were never alone and will not be alone as we face our challenging yet rewarding futures. We will be there to pick each other up when life gets tough and cheer each other on in the good times so that we can become the best physicians we can be.

From the Window
June 3, 2020

Thomas Amburn
University of Kentucky College of Medicine
Class of 2022

A RAINY DAY WHILE THE sun is out is a bad omen. But every day seems like a bad omen now. I stand by the window at times watching the strange weather passing through. If you look at the right moment, you will see me there with a face that mirrors the solemness of what I look at. The window glows with the lamp I have on, allowing its incandescent light to stretch along the walls. The hallway remains dark and silent. The barren solitude seems to have seeped in through the window.

Ambulances rush by my apartment in a periodic rhythm. It may sound bleak, but I often wonder who is in them and why. The sunsets have become more grey than usual despite the forecast calling for good weather. The rain taps its beat on the pavement below. I hear nothing else except a car passing by every now and again. Sometimes a bird sings out. Even that seems like a song of defiance during these times. We are not completely paused in this stillness but only moving at half speed.

I read stories of the breathless pandemic, but I see nothing with my own eyes. I am told it is everywhere, yet it hides every time I look. Our society has become scarce and returned only to our essentials, though I am still unsure of what those are. I thought that in serious times of urgency, a crisis would be immediate and evident. Yet after months of maybes and ifs, our speculations became reality despite no invitations of readiness.

Now the wind blows in through the window. Perhaps with it rides the rumors of terrible death and breathless fighting. But the streets outside remain quiet and the raindrops continue to fall. What am I supposed to think while hearing horrible stories yet seeing nothing at all?

The night time is the worst. Green lights from nearby houses shine along the roads wet from the rain. The traffic lights perform their show only for me now that the cars have nearly vanished. As if it were not possible, it is even quieter, the hallway even darker. Finally, the cry of the distant train breaks through the palpable immobility of the outside world. As quickly as it came, it retreats away.

I wonder what the neighbors across the street must be doing. Are they also watching from their windows? Looking for a sign or trying to regain their sense of normalcy? Will they look into my dimly lit window and wonder what I must be thinking?

These are times of wonder — not of magnificent landscapes or beautiful paintings but of tragedy hiding itself from so many of us. We attempted to set a timer, an end date that keeps extending forward as if running away from our useless grasps. No one speaks with surety anymore. Two weeks became a month, then two months, now possibly a year. Our crutches of time and agendas have eluded us, so we wait in its absence.

Plans have become broken sticks building only feeble structures. I try to disregard the situation that created the silence outside my window. However, each plan has been plucked away. Days trudge on, highlighting what I had planned on them. I planned a flight — canceled. I was set to take a career-defining exam — canceled. Canceled has become the word that gets my heart racing. I am completely powerless against its force as it traps me inside my apartment.

I have joined the latest trend — masks for the nose and mouth paired with concerned, distrusting eyes. I chose a simple, minimalistic black mask, but various colors and patterns are available to match individual preference. If you are lucky enough to get a hold of them, disposable gloves are the perfect accessory. These apocalyptic looks have become so normalized that it feels completely wrong to leave the house without them.

During my weekly grocery shopping, I measure with my eyes the length of six feet. The distances we keep from each other only intensifies the vacancy that roams our streets. A simple gesture of a smile has become elusive. The interactions that came so naturally before have been postponed. The solitude that has unleashed itself onto our streets now defines every aspect of our lives. The distances between us have swelled into expanses.

As I write into the night, the darkness continues to stare in through the window. We face each other as if in some twisted standoff, watching what the other might do. The rain has finally stopped, only accenting how quiet it is. The sirens of the ambulances still periodically rush by only followed by silence returning. These moments string along holding hands, one following another, stretching out time. I watch them slink by, one by one, expecting a final ending. My apartment has now become full of the eery solitude that squeezed inside between the cracks. I resign to wait in its mystery, half-expecting a sign from the window.

Step 1 in the Time of COVID

May 8, 2020

Paavani Reddy
Northwestern University Feinberg School of Medicine
Class of 2022

Apshara Ravichandran
Saint Louis University School of Medicine
Class of 2022

BEFORE MEDICAL STUDENTS embark on their clinical training, they must pass the United States Medical Licensing Examination (USMLE) Step 1. This year, like those before us, we entered our study periods for Step 1 with some trepidation — both about the long hours of studying and the high stakes of the exam. Like those before us, we reassured ourselves that if we put our time in now, we'd be able to move beyond memorizing minutiae to caring for patients in the hospital. And then, unlike those before us, testing centers across the world closed.[1]

The current significance of Step 1 in medical education cannot be overstated. Typically taken between the second and third years of medical school, Step 1 is the first of the many board exams that students must pass before entering residency training. A medical student's Step 1 score is one of the most important factors in their residency application and seriously impacts their future career opportunities.[2] In fact, most medical schools offer a six- or eight-week "dedicated" period during which students solely focus on preparing for this grueling eight-hour test. Between pre-clinical years when students are beholden to lecture content and tightly scheduled clinical years when they are beholden to clinical duties, these weeks are precious.

On March 11, the World Health Organization declared that COVID-19 was a global health crisis.[3] The National Board of Medical Examiners (NBME), which oversees Step 1, and the Prometric Test Centers, which administer Step 1, responded by closing exam centers on March 17 with plans to reopen in mid-April.[4] However, when the United States extended lockdown policies and individual states began operating on different timelines, many of us questioned whether reopening the test centers would be feasible given the proximity of students to each other while testing. Prometric extended closures twice more, doing so mere days before the test centers were to open. The most recent announcement stated that medical student examinations would begin May 1,[5] but scheduled exams would be subject to random cancellations to comply with state-specific social distancing guidelines.[6]

These delays may seem like a minor ordeal. However, many students were weeks or even days away from taking the biggest exam of their careers when the first round of closures occurred. Some had been in a highly-regimented "dedicated" period and suddenly were floundering. With no guidance directly from the NBME or Prometric, students began obsessively checking local government updates, refreshing testing site websites, calling test centers and scouring through speculative Reddit posts to piece together morsels of information.[7] Even the local testing centers sometimes offered different information than what was presented nationally. The newest wave of cancellations is keeping medical students guessing by potentially cancelling appointments at random less than 24 hours before their exam with no guarantee of later test dates.[8]

In tandem with these cancellations, Prometric has also opened new seats at test centers that don't seem to be open, leaving even students who never received a cancellation notice unsure if their test is valid.[9] To make matters worse, students still have to cope with the personal effects of coronavirus as well. Many students are immunocompromised, have ill family members or families financially impacted by the pandemic. Continuing to study as usual is nearly impossible.[10]

Scheduling adjustments are not only magnifying the stress of "dedicated" study periods for Step 1 but could also mean delays in students entering the hospital, engaging in research projects or contributing to student initiatives to directly address the pandemic. Due to a lack of testing sites and the random cancellations, many students who were slated to complete Step 1 before beginning their time in the hospital are now scrambling for test dates during their clinical rotations through different hospital services. This is inopportune when many students have used up thousands of dollars of practice materials, are already expected to devote substantial time towards rotation-specific exams (pediatrics, surgery, etc.) and may not have study time built into their third year.

As a result, some students are searching for testing locations outside of their local centers to find an open seat before they begin rotations. Because Prometric and the NBME have not implemented alternative testing methods, medical students will be driving or even flying across the country to take their exams. Those without the means to travel are left to either hope their local center doesn't close or to reschedule for a date months later — yet another manifestation of how medical school disproportionately favors the financially well-off.[11]

Complying with social distancing guidelines is a responsible action by Prometric and the NBME, but the temporary fixes that they are proposing took too long and do too little to address the impact of the pandemic on students. Delayed test center openings and appointment cancellations precede an inevitable backlog of exams for students who planned to take the exam in March, April and May — the usual test-taking months. Instead of continuing to push back tests in haphazard fashion, Prometric and the NBME could have looked at how other organizations that administer similar standardized exam delays have adjusted.

College Board, which oversees Advanced Placement exams, has maintained an active and organized website.[12] They are offering both free AP review lessons and remote administration of the AP exams taken by high schoolers for college credit. For the LSAT, the law school admissions exam, LSAC announced a plan to create a shortened, online-proctored LSAT-flex for students taking the exam in the near future.[13] The MCAT, the medical school admissions exam, will still be offered in-person, but to increase testing capacity, the AAMC is temporarily shortening the length of the exam and adding evening slots.[14]

Prometric could allow medical schools to proctor the USMLE Step 1 exam, or even send a Prometric representative to proctor these exams on campus. The NBME already administers secure national exams during clinical rotations at medical school campuses, which sets a precedent for on-campus testing. Alternatively, the NBME could hasten its pass/fail proposal set to be implemented by 2022 and modify the scoring of the exam during the pandemic.[15]

In the absence of pass/fail, for students anticipating how the emotional strain of a pandemic will affect their Step 1 score, perhaps statements from residency program directors would be helpful. For example, a move towards assessing the examination as pass/fail or through a more holistic and less numerical approach would go a long way towards showing humanity to students.

No one expects any organization to have the perfect solution to this crisis. These circumstances are unprecedented, and health care students make up a small portion of those affected. The NBME has made a few helpful gestures, such as releasing free practice exams and posting weekly updates (the latter, partially in response to an online petition).[16] They also recently released a statement noting their disappointment with Prometric's testing centers and added that they "are working hard to accelerate alternate test delivery solutions."[17] Still, this response comes after two months of vague, conflicting responses from the NBME and Prometric.

It is imperative that the NBME follows through on this statement in order to tackle the backlog in test-taking and the potential downstream effects for students entering the health care force in the next few years. On a more basic level, the current response shows a lack of compassion for how the pandemic has already impacted many students.

As one rising fourth-year medical student put it: "Let it be known that while med students have been told to adjust our expectations accordingly and have done so, nowhere has it been explicitly stated that the expectations of us will be adjusted accordingly." [18] Today's medical students will become tomorrow's physicians, and many are already stepping up to contribute to pandemic relief efforts.[19] We deserve the same respect and transparency from these institutions now as we will when we have "M.D." after our names. It is imperative that the NBME take this time to seriously reorganize and make big changes in this examination process, starting with prioritizing the primary stakeholders: medical students.

Silver Lining
June 4, 2020

Samantha M. Rodriguez
Florida International University Herbert Wertheim College of Medicine
Class of 2022

PEERING OUTSIDE TO witness an elderly woman walking her dog first thing in the morning — mask on, gloves on.

Passing by a beach normally teeming with families, lovers, life — now barren.

Riding bikes through the center of Coconut Grove, typically smelling of car exhaust and ethnic foods — now eerily devoid of traffic and human interaction.

A coronavirus — a positive-sense, single-stranded RNA virus as we have drilled into our memories — causing this void. Something so minuscule. Something invisible to the naked eye. The people of the world confined within the walls of their homes or a minimum of six feet away from another human being in a public space. So long as there are less than 10 people in the area. All due to this obscure villain of the world.

It almost seems unreal. The world has stopped as we anxiously await the "all clear" from some authoritative figure. The elderly woman continues reusing her mask and gloves as the store shelves have lacked stock for weeks. The beaches remain untouched. The busy streets are vacant. We have been halted in our tracks against all desires and efforts.

The world is quarantined, but we have learned to be human again.

Rather than tirelessly working or studying, we are forced to engage with one another in meaningful ways. We find novel alternatives to maintain relationships with those who mean the most to us during this daunting time with no foreseeable end. We reach out, check-in, virtually visit with our people. We adapt.

We learn to be children again. Playing board games, riding bikes, doing puzzles, speaking to friends on the phone without having a purpose for the call. We relearn the value of community, the beauty of nature, the joy in the triviality of everyday life. Life has come to a dramatic halt, but in this we find ourselves again. This does not negate the overwhelming stress and anxiety being experienced by the masses. It is only to find the silver lining in it all.

The silver lining of an elderly woman being able to safely walk her dog on empty streets.

The silver lining of a beach unfettered by plastic bottles and bags left behind by careless beachgoers.

The silver lining of a city street now free of pollutants, allowing for truly fresh air to fill the lungs of those who seek it.

The world is quarantined, but we are liberated just the same.

Lessons from Quarantine
July 28, 2020

Sylvia Guerra
Geisel School of Medicine at Dartmouth
Class of 2021

AS I WRITE THIS, more than 100,000 people have died in the United States from COVID-19 — more than any other country in the world.[1] The world has lost 358,000 souls. It seems both like yesterday and the distant past that I was last a learner in the hospital. Time now has a sense of meaninglessness that makes its passage difficult to mark, as days blend into weeks, weeks into months and so on.

COVID-19 was first confirmed in the United States on January 20 but didn't become a weather-like topic of daily conversation until early March. I was in the middle of a surgical intensive care unit rotation where I was busy falling in love with critical care. It was only slated to be a two-week elective, and that first week of 12-hour days was equal parts exhausting and exciting.

I remember working with one physician on the Monday of my second week who repeatedly mentioned how amazed she was that I was still allowed to be in the hospital every time that I asked a question or presented a patient. She even "offered" to send me home early that morning, but I declined, asserting that the school had yet to make any announcements. The email barring all students from clinical services came out that afternoon, and all medical students were sent home en masse.

The days that followed were filled with anxiety and sadness. How could they think that benching all of us was a good idea? I deep-cleaned the kitchen and living room. Don't we occasionally provide *some* value to patient care? I went for a run. Hasn't our training prepared us to be even *a little* useful? I started preparing for residency applications. What if we just worked with non-COVID-19 patients, so we didn't use up personal protective equipment? I reorganized my books. Isn't there *anything* useful we could do? I drank a lot of wine.

The truth is that I wasn't anxious about any of that. I was anxious because I was used to moving at such a fast pace that slamming on the brakes gave me whiplash. I was desperate for things to do because I had forgotten how to slow down and relax — how to just *be*. Slowly, I began to see the opportunity that quarantine had presented me with. We have all had to stop our lives, but having now had some time to think about the state of us, what parts of those lives do we want to take back up again once allowed to do so? What parts of our lives are better left in quarantine? And what really matters to us as members of society?

Quarantine was difficult at first because it challenged my identity. Who am I if I can't do the thing I've devoted myself to doing? Thinking back to medical school applications, I remember pouring my heart out onto the page and submitting *who I was* for judgment to the admissions gods who would decide whether or not I was worthy of entering the profession. I was judged to be adequate and was grateful to be given a white coat.

And yet, medical school itself has been a rather disease-like state. It has grown to take up space that didn't belong to it, metastasizing into every corner of who I think I am, eating away at self-esteem, relationships, and at some points, even my actual body. But my relationship with medicine is complex; it has also afforded me the enormous privilege of deeply connecting with patients at times of tremendous vulnerability and suffering as well as joy. Medicine has taken me to both the depths of my despair and to the heights of my humanity.

Being abruptly ripped away from such experiences in the hospital was painful at first, but having had a bit more time now to reflect, I can see that it was also healthy. This time in isolation has reminded me not only that I am more than a medical student; it has reminded me that my value as a person is inherent and not something I have to earn.

Slowing down has allowed me to see that I use productivity to try to convince myself of my own worth. On the days I've been "unproductive," I see myself as a disappointment, and yet on days that I accomplish a lot, I still don't feel good. Productivity feels like a baseline requirement. Where did this hungry ghost come from? The drive to be productive has convinced me that all time in which I am not producing something is somehow wasted and that the only way to feel better about who I am is to do more.

Unfortunately, I am not the only one who suffers from this disease. COVID-19 has exposed this at a national level too. In what other country do we see citizens protesting for their 'right' to produce and consume instead of their right to access health care so they can live?[2] COVID-19 has done a lot to expose a core American value: that productivity *equals* worth and that our value to society is commensurate with our ability to consume. I would argue that many of the deaths we've experienced in the United States have been caused by the deadly combination of both the virus and our consumerism. The "invisible scourge" isn't COVID-19; it's the way we dehumanize each other by valuing what we produce more than we value each other.

Perhaps the most important lesson I've learned in quarantine is just how valuable human connections really are. Truthfully, I think it is a deep instinctual knowledge of this fact that brought me to and keeps me in medicine. When I think back to the most meaningful experiences I've had in the hospital, I don't think of the days I was most productive and got the most tasks checked off my to-do list; rather, I think of the day I snuck off to my patient's room to celebrate her 88th birthday with a slice of carrot cake (her favorite) when her family couldn't visit. I think also of the day that I had the honor and privilege of holding my 55-year-old patient's hand as he passed away peacefully from a tragic accident.

The days I find most meaningful in the hospital are the days when, despite all else, the human connection between two people is most palpable — the days we are able to be entirely present with each other and experience joy or relief together. And I equally cherish those days when we face sadness and grief without turning away even — and especially — when it is difficult. Despite the ways in which medical training has been trying, I fall in love with it more and more each day.

As my time to return to the hospital approaches, I begin to worry that I'll lose the diagnostic clarity with which quarantine has allowed me to see myself and the 'diseases' that ail me. I wonder if I'll get lost again in the haze of productive busyness, losing the perspective I've gained in this time. But then I remember that each interaction I have with a patient or a colleague is an opportunity for connection, a shortcut back to this perspective that quarantine has given me. It's an opportunity to make meaning together and remind each other of our inherent worth, and no amount of busyness can get in the way of that.

The Pandemic

•

clinical

Should Medical Students Continue Clinical Rotations During the COVID-19 Pandemic?

March 17, 2020

Canon Brodar
University of Miami Miller School of Medicine
Class of 2021

AT LEAST HALF OF medical education is accomplished in clinical rotations where medical students learn the practice of medicine from supervising physicians. In recent days, some medical schools have canceled rotations in the face of a growing pandemic.[1] The halls of my own school have been abuzz with conversations of deans and students alike about how a medical school must operate during an outbreak.

In addressing some of these concerns, the Association of American Medical Colleges (AAMC) has recognized that students are "members of the health care team and can provide meaningful care," but schools may simply be unable to coordinate clinical experiences.[1]

Like many medical students, I am concerned about COVID and feel strongly that we ought to be on the wards.[2] As the AAMC acknowledges, medical students can contribute to patient care, and along those lines, there are good arguments that we ought to be allowed to do our part in combating COVID-19.[3] However, it is a fair concern that medical students staying home may help decrease the potential spread of COVID through social distancing, helping to "flatten the curve" and keep the number of cases below the health care system's capacity.[4] Regardless of which argument is more compelling, our effect as potential helpers or vectors is limited by the fact that there are relatively few of us compared to the massive numbers of essential or soon-to-be-essential medical personnel that will be needed at work in the coming months.

While we must evaluate risks and benefits of our options, our decisions about clinical education during a pandemic must be driven by an understanding of what it means to be a medical student. The coming months may be a defining moment for the U.S. health care system, and it will also be a defining moment for medical education. Are medical students learners, whose duty is to knowledge, or trainees, whose duty is to patients? I firmly believe that as a so-called "student-physician," my ethics ought to err on the side of physician rather than student.

For a physician, there is a clear and historic obligation to care for patients in the face of personal risk. The AMA Code of Medical Ethics states that "individual physicians have an obligation to provide urgent medical care during disasters. This ethical obligation holds even in the face of greater than usual risks to their own safety, health, or life." [5] As students, we do not yet have the power of our physician-teachers, and as such, many would argue that such obligations do not pertain to us. It is not just the power of physicians but rather their calling that demands such obligation.

Dr. Farr Curlin, a palliative care physician and a mentor of mine, taught me about such calling. He knows what the practice of medicine looks like when we reach the end of our ability to "fix" our patients. At times, the power of medicine fails.[6] When a physician provides care to the patient who cannot be cured despite the best effort of human technology and biomedical science, surely it is still medicine, and physicians are still obligated to care. Even still, there are times when a physician is limited in her ability to care, and there is nothing she can do but to be present with the patient in the midst of suffering.[7] Such moments reveal the calling at the heart of medicine: attending to suffering.

I cannot yet care or cure in the way that my teachers can, but I share this calling to attend to suffering. As a student who is not yet empowered to care or cure as my teachers do, my attention is often the best thing I can give, and it can even make a critical difference in care when I have the time and energy to discover a patient's needs that might not otherwise be communicated to my teachers. This call to attention will not disappear in the face of COVID-19. Instead, it will be amplified as a large portion of the population may suffer from the disease and its sequelae. Even though we medical students are not yet physicians, when the health care system operates at its capacity, our calling — and thus our obligation to care — should be even more clear. I only hope that our schools will allow us to step up and respond to it.

After all, this is what I signed up for when I entered medical school. I did not expect to learn medicine under only ideal conditions. On the contrary, as a medical student in Miami, I expected that I would learn medicine from some of the most vulnerable and remarkable patients that might need care in a U.S. hospital — many with tuberculosis, HIV, and any number of other communicable diseases that disproportionately affect our population. It will be my duty to care for such patients as a future physician, and if I do not learn now, when will I learn?

The AMA Code of Ethics has more to say about obligations during disasters, so that "when providing care in a disaster with its inherent dangers, physicians also have an obligation to evaluate the risks of providing care to individual patients versus the need to be available to provide care in the future." If we also extend this obligation to future care to apply to students, some will see grounds for keeping students off rotations out of concern for safety. Instead, I see it as an obligation to continue our clinical education for the safety of our future patients.

We who enter the field of medicine do so knowing that we may need to care for patients at the risk of our own personal health. We do not deny care to a patient with HIV or hepatitis C whose virus might be transmitted in the event of a needlestick. We do not shy away from the care of patients who have the flu or other infections that might lead to our own morbidity or mortality.

Regardless, based on the current evidence for the disease epidemiology, my classmates and I are at relatively low risk. According to the AAMC, the average age of U.S. medical students upon matriculation is 24 years old, and most students complete their program within four years.[8] Looking to Chinese data on COVID epidemiology, only 8% of cases occurred in patients aged 20-29, and only 3.8% of cases occurred in health care personnel.[9] The case fatality rate was 0.2% in 20-29 and 30-39 year old patients, and 0.3% in health care workers.[10]

If these disease trends hold true in the United States, the results may be disastrous to be sure, but as a healthy 28-year-old, I am not fearful for my own life and health but for the many patients who are at increased risk, namely those who are older or who have underlying health conditions.[11] These patients will experience lasting effects of the disease as will many others who may be triaged away from care as hospitals fill up. Today's acute problems will become chronic, and chronic problems left unattended will eventually become acute.

Such fallout of a global pandemic may last for years and will be compounded by looming physician shortages.[12] Next year's medical interns need to be ready for an overloaded system, to be prepared by a medical education that is adapted but not compromised. We will need the grit that comes from attending to our patients' suffering in the face of a pandemic.

Ultimately, this is the best argument for why medical students must be allowed to participate in clinical care: we must be ready for whatever comes next. Canceling rotations or restricting patient contact now will not suffice because the threat of COVID will not pass within weeks. We have already seen the disease affect China for months, and some reasonable calculations suggest hospitals could reach capacity in May or that a peak of new cases in the U.S. might only be reached by August.[13,14] If we do not continue training now, how will next year's physicians be adequately prepared to provide care in the future?

One of my professors, Dr. Jeff Brosco, likes to tell students that we have signed up for a profession that demands we run toward a fire and not away from it. We might just be students, but the direction that we run matters.

Medical Ethics in the Time of COVID-19: A Call for Critical Reflection

April 7, 2020

Adrian Anzaldua
University of California, San Francisco -
University of California, Berkeley Joint Medical Program
Class of 2021

AS WE ENTER THE fourth month of the COVID-19 crisis, stories of heroism from the frontlines of this global effort have been steadily forthcoming.

The first and most famous is the tale of Li Wenliang, the 34-year-old staff ophthalmologist at Wuhan Central Hospital. His advisory to colleagues on a private WeChat forum that a new SARS-like illness may have emerged and that they should prepare their families and friends eventually leaked to the global community. The alarm raised by Dr. Wenliang's accidental call to action won him an official admonishment from the Chinese government for "making false comments on the internet." [1]

After his passing on February 7 from COVID-19, the Chinese government rescinded the official admonishment and apologized to the late Dr. Wenliang's family. The people of the world are indebted to Dr. Wenliang's commitment to public awareness of the truth.

Miles away in Italy, the hardest hit European country to date, medical students are being fast-tracked into physicianhood nearly a year early. This quasi-conscription will free up seasoned outpatient providers who are desperately needed in emergency rooms and ICUs throughout that nation.

In times of crisis, we expect heroics of this sort from our physicians and physicians-in-training. As Canon Brodar wrote in his recent *in-Training* piece [page 21] calling for medical students to be allowed to train during this crisis, physicianhood, like the priesthood, is still considered a vocation by many: a profession whose practitioners are "called" to the work by a higher sense of moral purpose, if not by God himself ("vocation" from the Latin "vocatio" meaning "to be called or summoned").[2] This distinguishes health care workers from the vast majority of the modern American workforce, who wouldn't (or, at least, shouldn't) claim that their labor upholds a moral or religious obligation.

Our calling to care for the sick and suffering, regardless of their station or health status, is the moral engine that animates every inch of the American health care system. It is responsible for the everyday extraordinary actions of modern physicians. When our doctors stay hours after their shifts to see our sick children, when they spend days navigating byzantine insurance roadblocks to get us the right medications, or when they waive their fees when we lose a job or are just having a hard month, patients attribute these acts of kindness to the physician's moral calling to serve.

However, the world looks much different from the physician's perspective. What to a patient seems like an inspired act of goodwill is to the modern American physician an objective necessity of their work environment. Physicians and physicians-in-training go out of our way to provide care for patients not because we are better than anyone else or we feel duty-bound by a strict moral code but rather because we work in a system more dysfunctional than almost any other in America. So broken is the American medical system that without health care workers' myriad small acts of inspired goodwill, American patients simply wouldn't receive the ordinary, much less extraordinary, care they deserve.

During my first two years of medical school, I was trained in medical ethics just like all my peers, but I was also trained to recognize and respond to the social determinants of health that color so many of the medical problems our patients face. I was trained such that it is my duty to address the patient's COPD *and* their experiences of racism, poverty, housing insecurity and insurance status as it pertains to their health (which it always does). It is not enough to attend to a patient's biological pathophysiology; it is the interplay of biological, psychological, social, economic and political pathology that creates the symptoms and syndromes physicians treat.

I entered my clinical rotation year eager to bring this holistic view of medicine to bear on the patients I would have the privilege of working with. That all changed within the first month when I saw nearly as much suffering walking the halls as I saw in the hospital beds. The eyes of every provider were bruised by sleeplessness and fatigue. Providers called on the dark arts of gallows humor to alleviate their guilt for never seeing their husbands, wives, and children ("I bet I see my children even less than you do," I once heard one physician facetiously brag to another). One sees numerous "near-misses" and occasionally even a fatal error, unsurprising considering just how many patients our doctors are asked to manage simultaneously. In fact, medical errors account for approximately 250,000 deaths each year, third behind heart disease and cancer.[3]

In quieter, more inspired moments, my fellow providers would reiterate their own moral commitment to the holistic approach to medicine I was hoping to emulate as a student-physician. When we re-entered the fray after a quick lunch or spot of coffee, however, the stark realities of the practice of modern American medicine left little room for the exercise of morally-informed medicine.

Are we upholding our moral duty to the patient when circumstances force us to discharge a homeless patient with diabetic ulcers and heart failure back to the street? How about when we prescribe a necessary medication that the patient's insurance won't cover, leaving them to choose between life-saving medication and feeding their children? I hadn't expected that training as a physician would be nothing less than a trek through an endless moral minefield. After a few months on rotation I came to see cynicism and gallows humor as the scars of prolonged moral injury.

Medical students can't truly appreciate the bio-psycho-social toll that working in such dysfunction has on providers until they see it for themselves. The suffering among the licensed physicians was only half the story. As my clerkship year progressed, I witnessed my fellow classmates begin to take on the ego defenses of their higher-ups. The moral calluses showed more on some than on others, though everyone, including me, was forced to build up something of a thicker skin. Many people began dissociating to ease their suffering; others went for medication and therapy. No matter the method, all of us changed during that year on the wards — some of us into people who we had a hard time coming to terms with.

Having for the first time seen medicine for what it truly is and seeing how it affects its practitioners, I decided to take a year to study provider mental health and wellbeing and to help my school build up its student mental health infrastructure. In that time I came to understand that the failings of modern American medicine are best represented by the mental health crisis playing out in chart rooms across the country. The numbers are a tragedy.

According to one meta-analysis, American male physicians experience suicide at a rate 1.41 times that of the general population; female physicians at a rate 2.27 times the national average.[4] A retrospective analysis of resident physician deaths between 2000 and 2014 showed that overall, only cancer accounted for more resident-physician deaths than suicide; among male residents, suicide was the most common cause of death.[5] The prevalence of substance and alcohol use disorder, depression, anxiety and burnout among physicians far exceeds those of most other professions. On the whole, the American medical workforce is woefully unwell, thanks in large part to the fact that the moral center of American medicine has been under siege for decades.

So, as someone who's studied the moral, mental, physical and social havoc that the modern American medical system wreaks on trainees and providers, Mr. Brodar's invocation of moral duty is not the clarion call to action he believes it to be. To the trained ear, his call is an uncritical recitation of the ethical stance that, in our modern professional environment, has left providers vulnerable to injuries of all sorts.

Still, there are several reasons why I'm uneasy offering criticism of Mr. Brodar's position. First, his position is often taught in medical schools across the country, leaving those of us who disagree with the common stance feeling isolated and vulnerable as we enter the next phase of our career. Second, we are in a moment that truly requires medical heroics. Offering criticism of his position in the age of COVID-19 appears, at first glance, to be poorly timed. Third, and the most personal, I have always felt compelled by duty and have, on several occasions, "run toward the fire" as Mr. Brodar says we physicians are trained to do. To argue against him feels like disparaging my better nature.

Nonetheless, times of crisis peel back indifference and defenses to expose the true nature of things. The true nature of modern American medicine is that its practitioners were suffering through a mental and moral epidemic before the novel coronavirus ever arose. So when Mr. Brodar calls on students to "run toward the fire," he is encouraging them to run along a moral path so littered with hazards as to almost guarantee an injurious end, just as it has for many of those who have come before today's medical students. This type of uncritical absorption of expired ideals must not be passed onto the next generation of physicians whose job it will be to mend the moral mess we've inherited.

What's more, Mr. Brodar's evangelical adherence to the simplistic ethical dictates of our profession creates the conditions for confirmation bias on display in his own work. Yes, as Mr. Brodar noted, perhaps only 3.8% of Chinese health care workers contracted the virus, and perhaps the younger faired better than their older counterparts, but how many lives were impacted by those 3.8% becoming sick? Four percent of the NBA becoming sick doesn't matter but to the players and their families; 3.8% of the health care workforce becoming sick would have a tremendously negative impact.

This is before we even consider all the workers who would be forced to self-isolate when they find out their co-worker has been compromised by infection. The chance that a medical student could bring community-acquired COVID-19 into the hospital or outpatient clinic is too high a cost to justify continued learning, at least until we have better control of the current outbreak. Student utilization of precious personal protective equipment in a quickly worsening national shortage that is so bad citizens with sewing skills are being called upon to make medical masks is another cost to consider. How about the straightforward fact that medical student education draws time and effort away from patient care?

Do the potential benefits to medical student education justify all these grave risks to patient and provider health? Maybe, maybe not (likely not). Without a full rendering of the problem, there is no reason to have confidence in Mr. Brodar's simple moral arithmetic when more complex math is called for. In his zeal, Mr. Brodar has failed to show that medical student participation in this crisis would uphold the paramount ethical principle of medicine: first, do no harm.

However, if things turn for the worse, as they did in Italy, the expertise of advanced trainees may be called upon. When called upon, we will go because, at that point, it will be clear that our presence in the workforce provides a net benefit to all involved.

Though I disagree with Mr. Brodar's methods and conclusions on this issue, I do agree that this is an inflection point for modern American medicine. Our profession has been working at the breaking point for years, the costs of which have manifested as a mental health epidemic among our cherished providers and mentors. Only widespread heroism will keep our medical system from breaking under the weight of the COVID-19 crisis.

But when this chapter in medical history closes, it will be time for the next generation of providers to assume control over what is left. It will be up to us to build a medical system that doesn't rely on heroics for everyday functionality. Preparing ourselves for that responsibility is much more important and much more difficult than learning the specifics of providing care amidst chaos, especially when our presence could do more harm than good. If we're going to rise to the challenge of rebuilding our medical system to withstand the next crisis, medical students must critically appraise all aspects of our intellectual inheritance and let the full truth lead us where it must.

The Role of Third-Year Medical Students During the COVID-19 Pandemic
March 30, 2020

Matthew Henry
Wayne State University School of Medicine
Class of 2022

AS COVID-19 UPENDS domestic and international hospitals, it is also interrupting medical education. On March 17, 2020, the American Association of Medical Colleges (AAMC) and the Liaison Committee on Medical Education (LCME) jointly issued a statement supporting "medical schools in placing, at minimum, a two-week suspension on their medical students' participation in any activities that involve patient contact." [1]

The recommendation is unprecedented, as there is no evidence that medical students were pulled from clinical clerkships on a national scale during the H1N1 flu pandemic or recent epidemics such as Ebola, Severe Acute Respiratory Syndrome (SARS) and Middle East Respiratory Syndrome (MERS). The joint recommendation by the AAMC and LCME leaves thousands of third-year medical students, who will soon enter into their final year of school, contemplating their role in the face of this evolving pandemic.

What makes COVID-19, caused by the virus SARS-CoV-2, uniquely dangerous enough to temporarily pause clinical medical education?

First, the virus is extremely contagious. Epidemiologists quantify how contagious an infectious disease is with a variable called R naught (R0), which represents the expected number of cases directly generated by a single case. While data is still emerging for COVID-19, early estimates from the World Health Organization suggest the R0 of COVID-19 is between 2 and 2.5, meaning that on average every infected person will spread COVID-19 to at least two other individuals.[2] Comparatively, the seasonal flu R0 is slightly above one.[3]

Becoming infected with the SARS-CoV-2 does not necessarily mean a person will develop clinical symptoms of COVID-19. On the Diamond Princess, a cruise ship with infected passengers,[4] about half of the individuals who tested positive were asymptomatic at the time of specimen collection.[5] Although not all passengers were tested for the virus, using data from this cruise ship and applying statistical modeling, researchers estimate 17.9% of individuals infected with SARS-CoV-2 are asymptomatic carriers.[6] This data is important because asymptomatic carriers can unknowingly spread the virus, fueling the pandemic.[7] As such, social distancing is crucial to slow the spread of the disease.

In addition to being contagious, COVID-19 leads to significant morbidity and mortality. The case fatality rate (CFR), an epidemiological term representing the proportion of people who die from a specified disease among all individuals diagnosed with said disease, is between 0.25%-3.0%.[8] This estimated range is broad but still significant; the CFR of the seasonal flu is less than 0.1%.[3]

What is most concerning, however, is the stress that COVID-19 will put on our health care system. One analysis predicts 20.5 million Americans will require hospitalization with close to 4.5 million requiring intensive care unit (ICU) level care.[9] If the pandemic is concentrated to six months, this analysis predicts a capacity gap of about 1.4 million inpatient beds and 295,000 ICU beds. It is still early, and hospitals are already thin on resources: the Centers for Disease Control and Prevention (CDC) recommends using homemade masks such as bandanas and scarves as a last resort; some hospitals are converting operating rooms to ICU beds and others are using one ventilator for two COVID-19 patients.[10-12]

One would think that a health care system teetering on the verge of collapse would require all hands on deck, including physicians-in-training. After all, medical students play an important role in the care team: we coordinate care, speak with consulting services and case managers, explain confusing procedures and tests to patients and have time to spend with them and their families. Often, we are able to spend more personal time with the patient than the residents and attending physician on service.

However, everyday operations are disrupted in hospitals. The American College of Surgeons recommended postponing all non-high acuity surgeries;[13] medical students on surgical services are not spending time in the operating room but rather seeing consults, many of whom are in the emergency department. But some emergency departments are limiting student activity due to personal protective equipment (PPE) shortages. Medicine services are overwhelmed with suspected or confirmed COVID-19 patients, and as the AAMC previously stated, "It may be advisable, in the interest of student safety, to limit student direct care of known or suspected cases of COVID-19."[14]

In my experience on a neurology service, there were three patients awaiting COVID-19 results; it is safe to assume there are many more on internal medicine. For clerkships based in the outpatient setting, patients are no-showing or cancelling their appointments or the physician's office is rescheduling them altogether. This environment is not conducive to learning, which is the primary objective of medical students rotating on clinical clerkships.

Of course, people are still falling ill with other diseases during the COVID-19 pandemic, and they need our attention just as much as before. Some argue that medical students could assume more responsibility with these patients, allowing residents and attendings to focus their time and energy on COVID-19 patients.[14,15] This idea is fantastic in principle. However, we must humbly remember that all our clinical work is duplicated. Medical students do play an important role in the care team — but it is not vital. During this pandemic, it is crucial to limit patient contact with providers, as clinicians can serve as unintentional vectors.

There are over 20,000 third-year physicians-in-training at more than 150 medical schools in the country. Marc Lipsitch, an epidemiologist at Harvard School of Public Health, predicts at least 20% of the world's population could become infected.[16] Applying population data to third-year medical students suggest that about 4,000 third-year medical students will have COVID-19. Of these cases, about 700 would be asymptomatic carriers, potentially spreading the virus to other students, providers and patients. (These analyses do not consider that, as student-physicians, medical students are at higher risk of becoming infected.) Importantly, everyone in close contact to a student who tests positive COVID-19 would be required to self-quarantine for two weeks; students work closely with nurses, residents and attending physicians. The downstream effects of a student testing positive would further stress the health care system, and the risks do not outweigh the potential benefit we provide to the clinical team, at least at this time.

If third-year medical students cannot help in the clinical arena, then what is our role in the current climate? It is unclear, as information changes every day. Meanwhile, medical students can find creative ways to stay engaged, assist clinicians, and help our society better understand the disease.

We can educate our peers and parents about the importance of flattening the curve and that we are not immune to the risks of COVID-19 simply because of our age.[17-19] We can help collect and enter data and conduct initial analysis for research studies. During the Ebola outbreak, medical students were able to identify gaps in infection prevention in close to 100 facilities in a city in the Democratic Republic of Congo.[20] Blood is now scarce because thousands of blood drives across the country were cancelled;[21] medical students can promote awareness and encourage our peers to donate blood.

More directly, we could assist with triaging patients via telemedicine.[22] Already in progress across the country, students are coordinating babysitting and grocery shopping for providers on the front lines.[23] There are ample ways we student-physicians can help doctors on the front lines and our society as a whole while not putting patients and others at risk.

This pandemic is a rapidly evolving situation, and there might come a time when the benefit of deploying third-year medical students to the front lines outweighs the potential risks. COVID-19 patients will likely overwhelm the system, and many providers will become exhausted or stuck in quarantine. This problem is currently unfolding in Italy where the government is waiving the traditional graduation requirements and allowing thousands of student-doctors to enter the workforce eight to nine months early.[24,25] The National Health System in the United Kingdom is considering the same.[26] Now, Governor Andrew Cuomo of New York is calling on qualified medical and nursing students to assist, but their potential role remains unclear.[27]

The COVID-19 pandemic is quickly developing into disaster medicine at hospitals across the United States. During disasters, it is paramount that medical providers do not become victims themselves. Disaster medicine creates challenging ethical situations,[28] but the four basic bioethical principles — respect for autonomy, justice, beneficence and non-maleficence — still hold true.

First, we must do no harm. Having third-year medical students continue our core clerkships, where all our clinical work is duplicated, has the potential to do more harm than good. Nonetheless, we can contribute and play an active role in the COVID-19 crisis in unique and non-traditional ways. After the two-week clerkship hiatus concludes on April 1,[1] third-year medical students should not return to our rotations but rather be utilized in meaningful ways that help providers on the front lines.

Frontline
May 21, 2020

Maria Hanna
Northwestern University Feinberg School of Medicine
Class of 2022

Mask on.
Your own protective prison,
the air is stale but clean, you hope.
You don't dwell on things you can't change.

Check the morning news and choke
warning:
droplets filtered but rhetoric unencumbered.

Another day begins
wading into the fire wearing nothing but your robe
armed only with words of encouragement
chalked on the sidewalk in painstaking calligraphy.
You take up the sword,
but the blade is dull.

On the frontlines
you stand at attention
hoping to pass for the hero they call you
facing off against today's enemy:
the row of rooms marked "COVID+"

Each time you enter, you wonder,
to save a life
must you wager yours?

At 8 p.m. sharp,
the claps and cheers of thousands
ring out across the city,
but you don't hear them.
They fade beneath your patient's rattling lungs
drawing each breath as if questioning its worth.
Suddenly you hear only the hiss of your own breath
deafening, evanescent.

Finally home, peeling off layers
first sweat and grit
then scrubs
then skin.
You put on your new skin, the one that watches *The Office*
and bakes banana bread
and calls your family with a smile on your face.

And only when you have gone to bed
eyes closed, mind ablaze

Mask off.

The Pandemic

•

socio-legal

COVID-19 Lockdowns: Are They Legal?
April 15, 2020

Meghan Sharma
University of Miami Miller School of Medicine
Class of 2023

THE COVID-19 PANDEMIC has raised many questions about how to constitutionally handle a public health crisis on both the state and national levels. Many wonder if a national lockdown can be put in place — a new dilemma that has little legal precedent to follow.

Can individual rights be limited to protect public health?

Short answer: Under *Jacobson v. Massachusetts (1905)*, states may take measures to protect public health, even if it limits some individual rights.[1]

In the early 1900s, a smallpox epidemic hit the northeastern United States. When the epidemic hit Massachusetts, the city of Cambridge enacted a law that required all of its residents to be vaccinated against smallpox with a $5 fine of noncompliance. Henning Jacobson, a citizen of Cambridge, refused the vaccine and contested the fine, which ultimately led to the case reaching the Supreme Court in 1905. The court ruled that individual rights may be limited by the state for the purpose of protecting public health and that Cambridge's decision to fine Jacobson was just.[2]

This case, *Jacobson v. Massachusetts (1905)*, has set precedent that states may take action to protect the health and safety of its citizens, even if it may abridge certain individual liberties. Moreover, since this case is between a plaintiff and the state of Massachusetts, it specifically focuses on the state power, rather than the federal power, to address public health concerns. Although it is only one of many factors that play into the question of how to best protect public health while also acknowledging individual rights, it can help us better understand the current situation regarding COVID-19 in the United States.

Many states, including California, New York and Illinois, have taken statewide measures to limit the spread of the COVID-19 virus.[3] For instance, on March 20, New York Governor Andrew Cuomo signed an executive order mandating that 100% of the workforce must stay home, excluding essential services.[4] These measures enacted by states are valid exercises of power since states have the ability to take statewide measures in order to protect public health under Supreme Court precedent — precedent from *Jacobson v. Massachusetts*.

Is public health a state or national matter?

Short answer: While public health is traditionally under state jurisdiction, the federal government can become involved in several ways.

The issue becomes trickier when we begin to look at the ability of the federal government to impose national mandates during the COVID-19 pandemic, such as a national lockdown. Public health has traditionally been viewed as under state jurisdiction.[5] This state jurisdiction comes from the 10th Amendment of the Constitution, which says that any powers not delegated to the national government in the Constitution are reserved to the states.[6] Since public health is not explicitly mentioned anywhere in the Constitution, it is widely interpreted that public health is considered under state jurisdiction.

State governments may have more jurisdiction over public health than the federal government, but there are various ways for the federal government to get involved in protecting public health. For instance, the federal government may choose to evoke the Commerce Clause of the Constitution, which expresses that the federal government has the authority to regulate interstate commerce.[7] Thus, if a health crisis such as COVID-19 spreads beyond any individual states, the federal government may claim that they have the authority to prevent the spread of disease among states. This could allow for the federal government to take actions ranging from more interstate border screenings or potentially even a nationally mandated lockdown.

Another way that the federal government can influence health is through providing recommendations to the states. One of the main recommendations that the President has made during this pandemic has been the "stay-at-home" guideline. On March 29, President Trump extended the federal "stay-at-home" guidelines to April 30, stating that it is recommended that people stay at home until this date.[8] While this is only a "recommendation," many states have made decisions congruent with national guidelines.

How does declaring a "national emergency" change things?

Short answer: Declaring a "national emergency" can give the president and executive branch more authority over a situation such as the COVID-19 epidemic.

Laws and policies can — and often do — change during times of crisis.

Once a president declares a "national emergency," for instance, 100 special provisions become available for the executive branch to use.[9] Some of the most relevant provisions for a public health crisis include waiving confidentiality and certifications necessary to supply public health services and authorizing the use of unapproved drugs or devices.[10]

Moreover, courts and legislatures often defer more to the executive branch's decisions made during a national emergency. In this case, judicial deference may mean that the Supreme Court will defer more to executive decisions made on COVID-19 now that the issue has been declared a "national emergency." [11] This is all under the historical assumption that the president will act in the best interest of the country in times of crisis when there often is not enough time to go through the normal measures of getting actions approved by Congress.

COVID-19 was declared a national emergency as of March 1, 2020, which means we may see more deference towards the President's decisions in the upcoming months.[12] This is one of the few times that a national emergency has been declared due to a public health concern, as they are often for military or economic reasons.[13] Because of this, we may see new uses of national emergency powers within the next few months.

One of the most discussed actions the President has taken after declaring COVID-19 a national emergency was invoking the Stafford Act on March 13, 2020.[14] However, the Stafford Act was mainly intended for use during natural disasters, so its use for a public health issue has raised several new questions.

One such question has been whether the Stafford Act could be used to mandate a national quarantine, but it does not seem like the act itself could evoke a national lockdown.[15] The main intent of the Stafford Act is to enable the federal government to provide assistance to states and local governments through the Federal Emergency Management Agency (FEMA). This means that while the federal government can provide resources to states, it still cannot directly intervene in the crisis response of the states.

Can President Trump mandate a national lockdown?

Unfortunately, it is a hard question to answer. The COVID-19 crisis we face today is relatively uncharted territory in the legal realm. Not much legal precedent exists on how to respond to a public health crisis like this pandemic on a national scale.

There are many legal factors at play as well. Factors such as *Jacobson v. Massachusetts (1905)* and the Tenth Amendment may point to an argument that public health issues, including mandatory lockdowns, are primarily state concerns and that the national government should only be able to issue recommendations to the states during public health crises. However, if the President did choose to order a nationally mandated lockdown, other factors such as the federal power to regulate interstate commerce and presidential "national emergency" powers may help him in doing so.

With such little legal precedent, the decisions made in the next few months will be critical to better understand how both the state and federal governments should respond to public health crises.

Precedented: Historical Guidance on Freedom and Health in the Age of COVID-19

December 9, 2020

Adrian Anzaldua
University of California, San Francisco -
University of California, Berkeley Joint Medical Program
Class of 2021

UNPRECEDENTED. NO WORD HAS been used more often to describe this remarkable year.

At some point in the distant future, medical students of this era will recall being summarily removed from clinical rotations, uncertain if we would be asked to stay home or serve on the front lines of the fight against a global pandemic. We will recall when, during the summer of 2020, the moral and political duty to engage with the most momentous anti-racist movement since the 1960s reanimated a nation paralyzed by fear. By the fall, cataclysmic wildfires on the West Coast poisoned the air from San Francisco to New York City. Coronavirus, cultural upheaval and manifestations of climate change all bore down on us as we entered the most consequential and divisive national election in living memory.

As medical students we're taught to keep our personal politics out of the clinic. And yet, the nation's politics seep into nearly every aspect of medicine. The structural determinants of health that make our patients sicker and harder to treat are consequences of political decision-making; radical expression of political concepts like freedom and self-determination have dramatically worsened America's experience of COVID-19. Insofar as politics fundamentally shape how medicine is practiced, our responsibility to patients requires that we develop and maintain an expansive political consciousness.

With political consciousness-building in mind, the remainder of this essay will review the history of another period in American history defined by simultaneous struggle against government oppression and communicable disease: The American Revolution. Our review will expose the origins of American interpretations of freedom and self-determination. We'll end with a discussion on why political systems defined by a single, narrow conception of freedom are ill-suited to combat many modern public health threats and what we as medical students can do about it.

Before we begin our analysis, it's important to acknowledge that the lofty appeals to freedom that defined the American Revolution are invariably complicated by the period's malignant racism, sexism, and systematic oppression. The War of Independence was never meant to secure the Enlightenment principles of freedom and equality for anyone but White men. Keeping the period's intellectual contradictions and limitations in mind will help distinguish the period's problems and solutions from our own. With that caveat in place, let's turn to the events that laid the foundations for the political troubles we face today.

By 1775, many American colonists were fed up.[1] The American colonists understood themselves to be British citizens, entitled to the full rights and freedoms afforded them by law and custom. King George III and his government seemed to disagree when they failed to explicitly extend protections enjoyed by British citizens in Britain. To them, it appeared the colonies were unique entities, which entitled the Crown to keep a standing army stationed in cities up and down the Atlantic Coast during peacetime, even if the English Bill of Rights of 1689 expressly forbade such an action.[2] Besides, the young colonies had proven unruly; a standing police force might help keep things in order.

Police states are touchy. A slight bump here or an accidental nudge there can send matters spiraling out of hand. Such volatility helps explain why in 1770 a simple disagreement near the Boston Custom House quickly escalated into a violent confrontation between British soldiers and the townspeople, leaving five Bostonians dead.[3] The sentiments soured by the Boston Massacre would be further spoiled by the Coercive Acts, a series of laws that both robbed Massachusetts of its right to self-governance and kept British officials from having to stand trial in colonial courts.[4] Every British transgression, no matter how small, served to remind the colonists that they were not, in fact, protected by the rule of law as they were led to believe. To make matters exceedingly worse, colonists were being taxed for the privilege of living under imperial rule.

While many colonists held out hope for a peaceful resolution of grievances with King George III, Patrick Henry, a leader in the powerful state of Virginia, had enough. He made his sentiments known to delegates of the Second Virginia Convention late in 1775, offering a simple solution to the colonies' woes: raise a force of Virginians to ensure Virginia's defense.[5] Such a force would eliminate the justification for His Majesty's soldiers and the high taxes their presence demanded.

Henry's provocation sent the convention into a heated debate about whether such an action would invite war with the British. In defense of his resolutions, Henry delivered his now-famous speech with an ultimatum that grabbed the delegates by their spiritual collars and refused to let go: "Give me liberty or give me death!" A month later, a milestone in the fight to reform government according to Enlightenment ideals began in two villages north of Boston.

Just as the colonists took up arms to tear down the police state in which they lived, North Americans of all backgrounds began facing down a second, even deadlier enemy to freedom: smallpox. The variola virus, present in the Americas since Columbus's arrival in 1492, had chosen this particularly fraught moment to resurface in the British colonies of North America.[6] With no known treatments and an understanding that close contact with the infected increased the chance of falling ill, colonists implemented quarantine and self-isolation programs.

Some opted for inoculation (also known as variolation), a forerunner to vaccination that required inserting pus from a smallpox patient into an incision made in the healthy recipient's arm.[7] Variolation caused disease in the recipient, in some cases even leading to death. Despite these dangers, the prospect of immunity was enough to convince Abigail Adams to inoculate herself and her family.[8] George Washington reached the same conclusion for his troops after watching, helplessly, as the disease ravaged soldiers on both sides.[9]

Today, Americans once again find ourselves beset by the challenges of 1775. We are pushing back against the dual threats of police brutality and a deadly communicable disease in the midst of deep political division. Like a people besieged on all sides, attention to one threat raises the possibility of a sneak attack by the other. Our shouts of protest against police violence and systemic racism are muffled by the masks protecting our faces, lest we inadvertently invite the coronavirus into our lungs, then families, then communities. Despite a raging epidemic, Americans of 2020, like the colonists of 1775, have been left with little choice but to risk illness and violent ends in order to secure the full rights and freedoms afforded to us by law.

We are still years away from being able to fully reckon with the lessons of this year. Certainly, the events of 2020 have reinvigorated civic involvement. They've also reminded us that democratic politics and medicine take as their goal the same basic ideal: the enhancement of human freedom.

The overbearing nature of our current challenges might lead us to believe that our freedom depends on ridding ourselves of forces that restrict our freedom (i.e. structural and implicit racism, police violence, gross income inequality, climate change, coronavirus). This is what philosophers call negative freedom.[10] Those who advocate for small government do so for the same reason as those who advocate for police reform: fear that an over-empowered state is a threat to human freedom (and sometimes, to life itself).

While history is rife with justifications for building political systems to protect negative freedom, the costs of decentralized power become evident when a nation is met by challenges as harrowing as war or pandemic. Like an invading army, a communicable disease cannot be defeated by the uncoordinated, undisciplined effort of even a powerful nation, at least not without incurring incredible losses (Soviet losses during the Nazi invasion of Russia serve as a poignant reminder of the costs of being unprepared for a powerful enemy).[11] In order to push back against an adversary as powerful as coronavirus, the best of American ingenuity and will power must be organized and overseen by a government able and empowered to lead.

Yes, by empowering government in times of crisis we invite the possibility of future tyranny, but what sense does it make to invite significant, perhaps fatal injury now to avoid the risk of possible injury later? True existential challenges in the present not only warrant but demand that such risks be taken.

National emergencies like the COVID-19 pandemic help us see the shortcomings of building a political system too focused on limiting government power to protect negative freedoms. A significant portion of the nation is currently so suspicious of federal overreach that they would rather risk exposure to a deadly pathogen than invite the vague possibility of tyranny and oppression down the road.[12] However, if we don't give the government the power it needs to effectively organize the fight against COVID-19, we threaten not only the lives of fellow citizens but also the political economy on which we all rely.

Can we escape this dilemma with our health and freedom intact?

Yes, but only if we acknowledge the reality that certain problems cannot be solved by individuals and decentralized governments. As medical professionals who regularly deal with death and disease, we are well-positioned to advocate for balancing negative freedom with positive freedom, which means providing individuals the power and resources needed to manifest their will.[13]

How do medical students start down the road to becoming effective advocates for positive freedom?

First, and most importantly, by recognizing our position. As the incoming workforce for a profession desperately short on staff, our will, if expressed collectively, can reshape medicine into a force for the advancement of positive freedom. Second, students must organize and work locally. Get involved in your local chapter of White Coats for Blacks Lives, or find a community organization working with individuals experiencing homelessness or food insecurity. However you choose to develop your political consciousness as a medical student, be sure the experience requires you to intertwine some amount of your own well-being with the well-being of those suffering from the shortcomings of our political system. Consciousness grows when we have an emotional stake in the matter at hand.

Let's hope for our own sake and for our patients' sakes that the sacrifices of this year inch us closer to an America courageous enough to admit that a political system obsessed with negative freedom can itself be an enemy of freedom.

Cruel and Unusual Punishment: Incarceration in a Pandemic

June 15, 2020

Olivia Rizzo and Brianna Sohl
Wayne State University School of Medicine
Class of 2021

"I FEEL LIKE I'M IN a prison" is a sentiment that has been echoed as stay-at-home orders around the country have gained traction with almost every state in the United States having restrictions in place.[1] People are encouraged to minimize leaving their home to "flatten the curve" of the rampaging coronavirus disease 2019 (COVID-19) pandemic. It has been two months since COVID-19 was declared a pandemic.[2] People are itching to return to "normal," to break out of their so-called home confinement; however, what is it like to be a person in an actual prison right now, stuck in a crowded confinement that extends before and after this pandemic?

At the end of 2016, nearly 2.2 million people were incarcerated in the United States, the highest incarcerated population in the world.[3,4] There is a significant, disproportionate racial demographic wherein 2017 data illustrated that people who are Black represented 12% of the country but 33% of the incarcerated population.[5] Correctional facilities are functioning with more prisoners than the official capacity of the prison system is meant to sustain.[6] Approximately one out of every four people incarcerated is there due to nonviolent drug offenses.[7] Some people are incarcerated without actually having been convicted of a crime.[7] When it comes to the incarcerated population's health, one study found that 800,000 people who were incarcerated reported having a chronic medical condition, but they have limited accessibility to health care providers.[8] In fact, one physician from a Connecticut correctional institution disclosed that he was the only physician to care for 1,500 inmates.[9]

The Eighth Amendment of The Constitution states, "Excessive bail shall not be required, nor excessive fines imposed, *nor cruel and unusual punishments inflicted* [emphasis added]." In the 1976 court case *Estelle v Gamble*, the Supreme Court ruled that people who are incarcerated have a right to health care and that denying health care access or deliberate indifference to an inmate's health falls under cruel and unusual punishment.[10] Where then are we left as a pandemic floods through prison gates, putting all of those inside at risk? Additionally, when the tidal wave of this pandemic recedes, what will we as future physicians carry forward to serve those who experience incarceration?

The environment of correctional facilities — to confine all bodies within the same, limited space — is unsurprisingly a perfect incubator to facilitate contagious disease spread. This potential is compounded by other factors, such as bans on alcohol-based hand sanitizers, the transient movement of adults (approximately 7.3 million each year) in and out of local jails referred to as a "jail churn," and the staff of these facilities coming and going each day directly linking their local community to the residents of a correctional facility.[4,11] The consequences of this environment have played out with the spread of other infections such as influenza and tuberculosis.[11]

Even with anticipation of this potential, it did not lessen the loss when, on March 28, the first inmate in a federal prison died of COVID-19 complications; his name was Patrick Jones, a 49-year-old man in Louisiana serving time for a nonviolent drug offense.[12]

The Centers for Disease Control and Prevention (CDC) have published guidelines with recommendations for correctional facilities to mitigate the effects of COVID-19.[13] These guidelines include loosening restrictions on alcohol-based sanitizers, providing no-cost and adequate supply of soap for hand-washing and providing adequate communication to those who are incarcerated about COVID-19 risks, signs, and symptoms.

In conjunction with these guidelines within correctional facilities, additional advocacy efforts are calling for the active release of prisoners who are at higher risk for COVID-19 complications and who pose little threat to public safety.[14] Advocates state that this will aid in alleviating overcrowding within correctional facilities and protect people who are at higher risk of becoming infected.[15] Attorney General William Barr has released federal guidelines to help direct this process of decarceration.[15] As this process of decarceration continues, some argue that health care professionals should be at the forefront of this advocacy work, citing the field's ability to provide expert opinion, oversee release efforts and assess prioritization of prisoner release based on a comprehensive health screening.[16] With that being said, what is the role of medical students and medical education in our responsibility to the incarcerated population?

In general, as future physicians, we are not educated on the incarcerated population. We learn about rare diseases that affect only one individual in a million, yet people who are incarcerated represent 1% of the population and correctional facility health care is mystified. How often in our medical education do we learn beyond the health risks during incarceration, and understand how we as health professionals can support those who are incarcerated with transitioning into life after incarceration?[17]

In writing this piece, we acknowledged our own gaps that had to be filled to understand just how the incarcerated population is so especially vulnerable during the COVID-19 crisis. Small studies have shown what is intuitive to most: experiences working with and learning from the incarcerated population enhances the care future physicians can provide to those who have experienced or are currently experiencing incarceration.[18] Giftos *et al.* state, "While *Estelle v Gamble* established the legal right to health care for incarcerated patients in 1976, this right has not guaranteed access to clinicians with the knowledge, attitudes, and skills necessary to care for a vulnerable population in a complicated environment." [19] Perhaps our ignorance as physicians in training is not cruel and unusual punishment, but our complacency is at the cost of comprehensive health care that can and should be given to the millions of people who experience incarceration.

The outbreak of COVID-19 has magnified the fact that those experiencing incarceration are intimately tied to our society and community. It is our job as future physicians to choose to pay attention and make concerted efforts to not turn a blind eye toward people who are incarcerated as is frequently done by society. People who are incarcerated are entirely at the mercy of their institution as to how they are protected and medically treated. Someday we will be the physicians given the opportunity to deliver compassion and care to those individuals. Some of us will see these patients in the inpatient hospital setting for an urgent surgical procedure during their incarceration, or in a maternity ward when a person who is incarcerated is in labor, or in a primary care clinic for an annual physical months after they have been released from incarceration.

Now more than ever, we must recognize that society is intertwined no matter the geographic, political or physical boundaries. The boundary between those who are incarcerated and those on the outside is porous. If we want to be better prepared for the next pandemic and be better prepared to treat and serve our future patients, we must realize that COVID-19 is exacerbating pre-existing issues in correctional health care. It is up to us to take advantage of this opportunity to cultivate a culture which underscores the importance of correctional health care in medicine.

THE PANDEMIC

496 Beds: Medical Students Call to Action
May 1, 2020

Hannah Roach at Lewis Katz School of Medicine, Class of 2024
Kristin Spiegel at Drexel University College of Medicine, Class of 2021
Jenny Nguyen at Lewis Katz School of Medicine, Class of 2021
Emma Schanzenbach at Drexel University College of Medicine, Class of 2021
Natalie Marie Dicenzo at Drexel University College of Medicine, Class of 2020

WHY IS A HOSPITAL standing empty? As dust gathers across abandoned wards, 496 beds lie empty. Amidst a growing pandemic, Philadelphia scrambles to accommodate the 12,566 cases of the novel coronavirus as of April 27, 2020.[1] As numbers continue to rise and the city treats patients from the nearby epicenters of New York and New Jersey,[2] the recently-closed Hahnemann hospital could alleviate this bed shortage.

Hahnemann historically served as a safety-net for the city, providing care for a majority of Medicaid and Medicare patients, until its new owner Joel Freedman, a California-based investment banker and CEO of a private equity firm,[3] filed for Chapter 11 bankruptcy in 2019.[4] Hahnemann had been experiencing 14 straight years of financial losses under its for-profit model,[5] and even with state and city efforts for financial contribution,[6] the hospital was ultimately deemed too expensive to save. The hospital closure allowed Freedman the opportunity to liquidate its assets,[7] including valuable Center City real estate. Despite efforts by community members and providers at the time, the closure of Hahnemann left behind Philadelphia's most marginalized and vulnerable populations.

This is not the first time that Philadelphia has faced a pandemic nor the first time shuttered hospitals have been required to meet demands. During the Spanish Flu epidemic in 1918, Philadelphia was one of the hardest hit cities.[8] The Medico-Chirurgical Hospital,[9] which had been closed to make way for construction of the Benjamin Franklin Parkway, was emergently reopened by the City and its medical schools. History has come full circle in Philadelphia; patients are once again in desperate need of beds, and the city is aiming to restore institutions once condemned.

This time, the city was faced with an impossible decision: to purchase the building from Freedman or lease for close to $1 million a month.[10] Freedman and his group believe they are accommodating the City by asking for a reasonable price. Meanwhile, Temple University has offered the Liacouras Center with 250 beds free of charge.[11] However, this is just half of what Hahnemann has to offer. While Mayor Jim Kenney denied the City's need for Hahnemann and stated that negotiations are over,[12] Philadelphia health professionals remain desperate for bed space.

Our United States government just printed $2 trillion to save small businesses.[13] So why do 496 hospital beds lay empty? We believe the City of Philadelphia should seize Hahnemann from Freedman and abolish any private ownership of a hospital in times of crisis.[14] The value of human lives are not priced per bed.

Holding Hahnemann Hospital hostage in the context of a global pandemic prioritizes profits over people. At the time of Hahnemann's closure, other hospitals in the city wondered how they would absorb the additional patient volume without compromising quality or safety.[15] The scale of this pandemic now makes one thing very clear: there are not enough hospital beds in Philadelphia to care for everyone who will be infected. The city may not see the peak of the epidemic until June,[16] and it is uncertain if the city's hospitals will have the capacity to support its citizens and the patients from overburdened New York City and New Jersey hospitals.[17]

This isn't a problem that only affects Philadelphia, but one that every city may soon face.[18] And while we all must live with this virus, we are not affected equally. We are not affected equally when over 10 million people filed for unemployment in March 2020.[19] Not when health care providers are dying because of unsafe conditions without proper PPE.[20] Not when Americans are reluctant to go to the hospital due to a lack of medical coverage and must choose between potential death or a $10,000 bill.[21,22] Many of the essential workers we now tout as heroes may not even be able to afford coverage.

This country must come face to face with our broken health care system, of which Hahnemann is a prime example. Operating health care as a business model, as CEO Joel Freedman did, is unsustainable. We call for an America with universal access to health care, and that requires hospitals where such health care can be administered.

In a society where the government and infrastructure have left us unprepared, we as civilians are all on the frontlines. All community members have the agency to make decisions that will influence the spread of the pandemic, but individuals with tremendous wealth like Freedman have an opportunity to redistribute their resources for the greater good of entire communities. Now more than ever calls to question a for-profit system that serves to benefit the shareholder. Now more than ever there is a call for health care for all.

Hahnemann's doors stay closed and our patients are waiting. While Philadelphia has stopped negotiations, we, as students with futures in health care,[23] cannot accept this. We are organizing to help mitigate the crisis even as we are sidelined, but it is not enough. We demand that Freedman provide free use of Hahnemann for the duration of the pandemic. If he does not comply, we demand that the City of Philadelphia and the State of Pennsylvania invoke any and all emergency powers necessary to seize and reopen the hospital. We have 496 beds waiting. We call on the people of Philadelphia to take control of our own future and help us secure the hospital as a space to save lives rather than bend to the will of multimillionaires like Freedman, who contribute to a system that works for shareholders and not the patients. We, the people of Philadelphia, can build a better one.

Now is the time to ask Philadelphia to live up to its name.

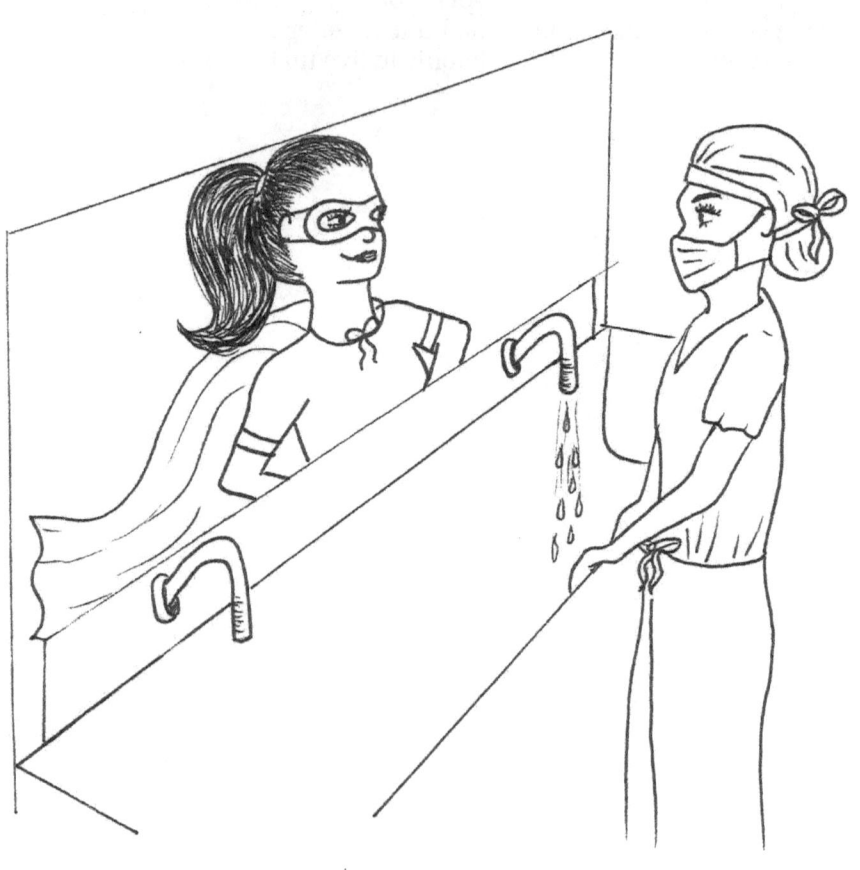

Intimate Reflections

•

inward

A Nation On My Shoulders
November 26, 2020

Neha Deo
Mayo Clinic Alix School of Medicine
Class of 2023

Failure was never an option for me.

Every time I fail
I am reminded that I have let my country down.

My ancestors, who worked as slaves in the sugarcane industry
on an unfamiliar island.

My grandfather, who passed before reaping the fruits of his labor
in an unfamiliar country.

My parents, who worked as immigrants to make ends meet
on an unfamiliar continent.

In failure I disappoint a community,
a country,
that rests on my shoulders.

My ancestors' blood runs through my body
and this serves as a reminder
that I cannot surrender.

Lessons on Coronavirus From My Great Grandpa Saul
May 6, 2020

Samantha Greissman
University of Miami Miller School of Medicine
Class of 2020

GREAT GRANDPA SAUL Matelson was a family physician living in Brooklyn, New York. He did it all: mended bones, delivered babies and treated infections. In 1983, at the age of 77, he underwent surgery to repair a colonic perforation and required a blood transfusion. Unbeknownst to him, it was infected with the human immunodeficiency virus (HIV).

Five years later, Saul presented to the hospital with profound diarrhea and painful mouth sores. Upon arrival to visit their father, my grandmother and her sisters were surprised to see that he had been placed in isolation. Confused and frightened, the Matelson sisters stood outside Saul's room while an infectious disease doctor told them that their father had acquired immunodeficiency syndrome (AIDS).

All four were horrified to learn that Saul had a "gay man's disease" and decided not to tell him or anyone else. They fed him a number of lies, including that he was just suffering from a cold and would eventually recover as well as that he was bitten by a mosquito on a trip to South America, contracting an untreatable disease. Saul's daughters rarely brought him to see doctors, and physicians never made home visits. So he knew whatever was wrong must have been incurable. He was convinced it was cancer.

But something didn't add up. Families of cancer patients don't regard their loved ones with disgust. Despite Saul's pained, lonely eyes, my grandmother feared his "dirty blood" and avoided coming in contact with him. She refused to use the bathroom in his apartment or kiss him 'hello' and 'goodbye,' a decision she now lives to regret.

Long before I knew this story, I began inadvertently building a career in a field deeply connected to Saul. As a child, I became interested in physician "microbe hunters" in novels and on television. Throughout high school and college, I pursued volunteer opportunities to study infectious diseases and eventually earned a master of public health in infectious disease epidemiology. Unsurprisingly, my passion manifested itself in medical school with infectious disease research and electives. Among my peers, I am the "infectious disease girl."

Through all of these experiences, my grandmother resisted my passion, unabashedly voicing her disapproval. "Ain't there anything else you're interested in?" she would ask in her thick Brooklyn accent. "I don't want you around those needles!" The reason behind her disapproval remained a mystery to me. It bothered me though, and I repeatedly found myself on the defense about my aspirations. I always thought that having a granddaughter studying to be a doctor would satisfy my Jewish grandmother's pride. But she seemed disappointed.

I finally learned the truth about Saul during my second year of medical school. As we sat in the car on the way to dinner — grandma, grandpa, mom and I — she attacked my passion for infectious diseases yet again. Until suddenly, grandma spit it out. As the story rolled off her tongue, I could barely catch my breath. I wanted to travel back in time to be with my family during this tragedy as someone who could properly explain Saul's diagnosis. I wanted to break down the barriers they constructed between their love for Saul and his disease. As I sat in the backseat, it dawned on me that I was unknowingly training to be a physician who could have treated Saul.

I'm grateful that we now live in a world where the science of HIV transmission is better understood, increasingly chipping away at social stigmatization. Graduating medical school amidst a terrifying coronavirus pandemic, I recognize that I am about to enter the health care workforce during my generation's version of the "HIV scare." We must carry over important lessons from one pandemic to the next.

Before Saul was sick, it was a tradition that the sisters would kiss their father 'hello' and 'goodbye' when he left for and came home from work. When he retired in South Florida, this practice continued when they visited his oceanside apartment. One day, they just stopped. It would be naïve to think that this went unnoticed by Saul, whose career depended on recognizing patterns that point toward diagnoses. In infectious diseases, isolation becomes both the greatest tool and the most punishing weapon. In the HIV pandemic, my great grandpa Saul died isolated from his family, who viewed him as a walking fomite. They feared his disease and "protected" themselves from contagion. AIDS may have been the direct cause of Saul's death, but the abandonment by his family resulted in a critical insult to his human spirit.

There are miles differentiating the circumstances of social distancing between HIV and COVID-19, but the effects remain similar. Today, my grandparents are older than Saul was when distanced from his family. Now during the coronavirus pandemic, they too are isolated. This time it's not because they are the fomites, but because I might be. Those big enveloping hugs that grandma lives for and kisses from grandpa will likely become a thing of the past.

As we enter a new world that discourages contact with the aging population, great grandpa Saul's story reminds us that we cannot let them go through this alone. Call your grandparents, parents and elderly loved ones every day. Give them some form of human connection that inspires them to look forward to every new sunrise. While we all practice social distancing for their protection, it is they who most bear the burden of loneliness during the coronavirus pandemic.

Soon I will start an internal medicine residency at Columbia-New York Presbyterian Hospital and move back to the city where great grandpa Saul flourished as a physician. Now the same city is unrecognizable following the outbreak of COVID-19. My grandmother's worst fears of me being exposed to infectious dangers are coming true. During our daily quarantine video chats, she never fails to warn me of the number of COVID-19 cases in New York. From these conversations loaded with concern in my grandma's voice, I realize now that my career choice never disappointed her. Rather, it worried her.

We've come a long way as a family scarred by HIV's worldwide devastation. I've taught my grandmother about HIV transmission and personal protective equipment. She listens to me when I say that she should not leave the house right now. In return, I collect her list of groceries and drop them off at her home in South Florida. We sit at least six feet apart on the driveway, my grandparents on folding chairs in the shade of their garage. After talking for an hour or so, I remind them to wash their hands when they go back inside. When we video chat over dinner later that evening, they say that my visit was the best part of their day. Then, they inevitably ask for the hundredth time when I plan to head up to New York. "Make sure you have a mask!" grandma so helpfully reminds me.

At this point, it's clear from our conversations that my grandmother accepts that infectious diseases are my passion and future career. And on my end, I've accepted that some things will never change. A worried grandmother will still always be a grandmother.

three machines
October 15, 2020

Kirsten Myers
University of Washington School of Medicine
Class of 2023

i come from:
not white coats and stethoscopes,

> "I saw three red-tailed hawks the night before my wife died
> I took that as a good sign.
> They asked me if I wanted her to do the operation

empty churches
with art-deco stained glass,
no preacher, no pastor, no doctor,

> I couldn't go to sleep that night until 2 a.m.
> but I thought we had two doctors telling me to go ahead
> and they must know what to do"

where people disappear
diagnosis never known
the only consult: prayer.

> "She passed on twice during the operation"

i sit a stranger,
in lecture halls,
in patients' rooms,
in exams,

> *"Her heart stopped.*
> *The third time they brought her back to life*
> *she was kept alive by three machines.*
>
> *They asked me what I wanted to do and*
> *I said her living will didn't want her to be*
> *kept alive on three machines."*

so one day
i can translate to my patients
what my family missed.

> *"She's the first one in our family that wants to be a doctor*
> *and I'm proud of her."*

CLL (Child Learning Love)
September 10, 2020

Gabriel Davis
SUNY Downstate College of Medicine
Class of 2022

Chanukah

Latke grease and shrinking blue candles —
The nostalgia invisible because you still haven't told us.
This year my gift to you is being an ass, for I am
The Son who Needles. But my latest taunt
Lights new flames of hurt in your eyes, and I know immediately
That something is different now:
You say, *You will miss me when I'm gone.*
You mean, *I am sick, and you have taken me for granted your whole life.*
Your voice is hot with oil and the dark wisdom of elders.
I remember that the miracle of Chanukah is a children's story.

Yom Kippur

You call me on a Thursday to tell me
You were diagnosed with leukemia in October.
I put on my medical student cap and ask about
Biomarkers. Every year on Yom Kippur
I try to remember the sins I've committed.
But this year, beneath the cleansing saltwater of my tears,
I finally remember all of the small, terrible things I've done to you.

Passover

We haven't seen you since you told us, and
We haven't had a family *seder* since we left for college;
But this year we brothers conspire with
Kind intent at last. So when you walk into The Den
To find us all Home, unannounced, and when you finally
Let the sobs from which you'd always protected us
Buckle like crashing waves from your strong, tired face, I remember
The fierce, imperfect blood that once filled your ancestors in Egypt,
And now fills you, and even your children; and I remember
The Red Sea you held open for us
Just long enough.

— For my mom

IN-TRAINING: 2020 IN OUR WORDS

Pattern Recognition
January 30, 2020

Samantha Schroth
Northwestern University Feinberg School of Medicine
MD-PhD Trainee

IN MEDICINE, YOU learn to recognize patterns. An elderly patient presents with shortness of breath and lower extremity edema: add heart failure to the differential. A young African-American female reports a dry cough and difficulty breathing while walking to work: consider sarcoidosis.

These patterns often provide a helpful service, aiding in the assimilation of a tremendous amount of knowledge that must occur as one progresses through medical education and training. The recognition of their existence and subsequent use is typically rewarded — a readily available response when the chief resident asks for a differential diagnosis of the newly admitted patient with severe back pain and vomiting; another correct UWorld question; a higher score on a career-defining exam.

However, what happens when the patterns we've learned to recognize are an inaccurate representation of reality? What happens when we begin accepting patterns portrayed in the media and our social networking sites as fact?

Although I've spent only a mere two and a half years as a student in this world of medical education, it's readily apparent that I fit into very few of the "typical medical student" patterns. I'm part of a small cohort of dual degree students. I'm nontraditional, having never considered becoming a physician until after I graduated from college in 2013. And I am a disabled woman.

Making such a statement — "I am disabled" — typically results in a shift, a turning of the tables, as you must now decide how or if that changes the way you receive the words of this writing.

I spent the majority of my life seamlessly fitting into the world around me until a freak accident and a falling dead tree changed everything. Abled to disabled, walking to wheeling, I slowly discovered the patterns that had been deeply ingrained in my own mind about the value of my now disabled self-worth. These patterns have also been imprinted on my fellow classmates, professors and future patients.

Paralysis has added an additional label to my demographic identity, just as it has added an additional lens to my view of the world. This lens, while sometimes worn with tears and frustration, has provided clarity and acknowledgment of an earlier perspective I once held. A perspective where implicit bias built on poorly informed patterns ran unencumbered, further propagated by ignorance and "not my problem" thinking. A perspective where individuals with disabilities weren't viewed as equals and never could be.

I will forever remember holding onto a closed envelope from the DMV, the weight of which seemed infinitely greater than the blue and white placard it enclosed. A new marker to hang in my vehicle, a new identity to accept, a new reality I was forced to inhabit. And yet...

My life has continued along its path, albeit a rather different path than my previously intended journey. I certainly have my fair share of struggles, but my accomplishments, many a direct result of my injury, speak for themselves. Outside of pursuing a career as a physician-scientist, I race marathons using a specialized racing wheelchair and have qualified for the Boston Marathon twice. I've served as Ms. Wheelchair Wisconsin and Ms. Wheelchair America, advocating for persons with disabilities on a national stage. Six years since my injury, I live my life with passion and pride using my wheels to propel both myself and my goals to fruition.

The patterns our society has come to associate with disability — incompetence, inferiority and expectations of a life of misery — are not the reality. In allowing acceptance of these ignorant and fallacious patterns, we create barriers that deter and deprive, allowing doubt and self-loathing to shroud the mind of a newly injured patient or fear to overwhelm soon-to-be parents receiving news of an extra chromosome.

As trainees, educators and physicians, we possess a unique ability to impact the lives of others in profoundly influential ways. Recognizing the source and addressing the reliability of the patterns we use to inform our actions and reactions is therefore not only important but imperative as we interact with countless individuals that possess experiences vastly different from our own.

Patterns exist.

Recognize them for what they truly are, no more and no less.

My First Stitch: A Dramatic Retelling
June 24, 2020

Eric Bethea
Emory University School of Medicine
Class of 2022

"COULD YOU PLEASE HAND Eric the needle driver?" As the scrub tech loaded up that blessed golden tool, I knew that I had just ascended within the realm of surgery. Last week, I had been nothing more than an unusually talkative pair of retractors. Now I had become Eric, the one who could close skin incisions of "very short" to "moderately short" length.

I took the tool in my hand with great pride and thanked the scrub tech in my most confident tone. She peered out at me from over her mask, congratulating me with her eyes. She understood what had just taken place.

The incision was approximately two centimeters long, and it was up to me to bring the edges of skin back together as God intended them to be. I felt the weight of the responsibility weighing on my shoulders, which were already sore from standing completely still with my arms fearfully tensed for the past four hours. I ran through the arsenal of stitches I'd been taught and realized that there was really only one with which I could claim any degree of proficiency: the subcuticular stitch. This sacred technique was passed down to generations of medical students around the globe to help them survive their surgery rotations. Today, it would be my saving grace.

I looked back down at the incision and began planning my approach. It had been used as an entry for one of the ports in the laparoscopic surgery that we (they) had just completed. Approximately three-or-so centimeters below the costal margin in the patient's left upper quadrant, I visualized all of the adjacent structures in my mind's eye. The spleen and its associated vasculature, the left hemidiaphragm, and the gastric fundus were all the vital structures I knew I would need to keep in mind as I attempted to stitch the patient's subcuticular tissue back together. There can be no mistakes and no overabundance of caution in the operating room.

INTIMATE REFLECTIONS

After I completed my analysis, I realized that the resident opposite me was suturing some of the last few port sites on his side. I clenched my hand on the needle driver in frustration: time was running out. The eyes of the OR would soon be upon me.

I began my approach, firmly but carefully lifting one side of the wound as I had practiced tens of times before on pig skin in my training leading up to that moment. I set the anchoring stitch in place and pushed along.

The first dip of the needle into the skin was perfection. Its sleek metal body slid gracefully through that delicate line between the dermis and epidermis like an Olympian diving into the water without a splash. I let out a sigh of relief. Unfortunately, my reprieve proved to be short-lived as I heard the familiar crack of Dermabond, a medical adhesive, being prepared for application. My resident had finished closing the other sites. If I didn't complete the stitch now, I would have to face the scrutiny of six pairs of eyes all trained on my hands. I would be the last obstacle keeping everyone from the few precious minutes of break time we had between cases.

I reloaded the needle and took a bite on the opposite side, making sure to roll my wrist as was my tendency to forget. As easily as the first, the needle slid through the dermal-epidermal junction and exited inside of the wound. I could hardly contain my excitement. Everything was going according to plan.

"Looks good Eric," my resident said to me, who had taken to observing my work. "Now tie it up and let's get out of here."

My heart sank. The blood in my arteries ran cold. My hands floated impotently in the air. The accursed tie! I thought back to those days in the simulation lab when I would look down at my horribly disfigured ties and assure myself that it would all come together soon enough. How could I have been filled with such hubris? Now it was too late. Fate was to claim my good fortune as it does for all prideful men.

"You can do a hand tie or an instrument tie, whichever you know how to do," my resident stated. Alas, I pleaded with my eyes, therein lies the issue. What little I had known about either technique had flown from my mind. My brain had been wiped with mental chlorhexidine, killing 99.9% of intelligent brain activity. I stood frozen with either side of the suture in my double-gloved hands. Before I could formally give up, panic set in and my hands began pantomiming the motions for tying a knot, like a toddler who had just been handed a pair of shoestrings. Witnessing my struggle, the resident took pity on me.

"Here, let me help you with this one," he said. "We can talk it over afterwards, and you can try again in the next case."

I nodded. My composure was cool on the outside, but on the inside, I was devastated. I had disgraced myself, my family, my medical school, and the human race all at once. There was no way I was going to recover from such a B-team performance, I thought to myself. I was beginning to spiral into despair when I heard a voice call my name. It was our scrub tech. She was smiling at me.

"It's okay," she said. "Everyone has trouble with their first few. It's no big deal. You'll get the next one." I smiled back at her and laughed weakly.

Those were the exact words that I needed to hear in that moment. Thank God for her. I knew she was right. As we began wheeling the patient out of the room, my body began to unclench, and the onslaught of anxious thoughts slowed. I immediately began planning the approach to my next port closure with my newly freed mental space. As we went down the hallway, I imagined my hands positioned over that damn two-centimeter incision like a trained athlete visualizing his next in-game performance.

Next time, I would be ready.

Intimate Reflections

•

outward

Buddy
October 5, 2020

John Carlo Pasco
Boston University School of Medicine
Class of 2021

"YOU CAN'T LIE TO a liar," you said, but in more colorful terms. You were sitting up in your bed and I had just interrupted your breakfast. "You can't lie to a liar, so just tell me the truth, Doc. What's going on?"

You were my first patient on my first inpatient rotation as a third-year medical student, which meant that I had absolutely no idea what was going on. I was mostly concerned with trying not to faint during presentations on morning rounds. I stared at your bowl of Cheerios, the cereal beginning to turn the skim milk a pale yellow. Your brow furrowed in annoyance behind your thick glasses.

I tried to put your story together in my head: you came to the hospital because your skin was yellow — not white like it should have been — and your urine was brown — not yellow like it should have been — and your stool was white — not brown like it should have been.

I did not know what was happening. I felt exactly how I'd been trained to feel when I didn't know the answer to a question: I felt I was failing you. But I promised I wouldn't lie to you.

"I don't know," I admitted, "but based on your story, I'll suggest some tests to the whole team taking care of you. Whatever is happening, you and I will figure this out together." Legally, I felt compelled to add, "And I'm not a doctor yet, I'm still a medical student."

You chuckled, "Okay, buddy." Your brow softened, relaxed into the face that I would come to know over the next month.

When I learned about jaundice in medical school, I concentrated on the mechanism, the risk factors, the potential causes, the lab values. I learned to look for subtle yellowing of the skin and sclerae on the physical exam. I was wholly convinced that I would never appreciate these changes in skin tone.

The bilirubin I imagined depositing in your skin did not turn it an artificial yellow like I had naively envisioned; instead, it blended naturally with your complexion, highlighting certain parts of you. I saw your face, with skin like aged parchment, into which vignettes were brusquely etched. I saw through your thickened lenses, which magnified your eyes like two movie screens showing old war movies in tones of sepia and amber, projecting unspoken sights from Vietnam. I saw your palms, rough with callouses, and when I shook your hand at the end of our interview, I felt that those flaxen patches sought to tell a story, but I was still learning your language, too blind to read it yet.

"We'll just take this one day at a time then," you said as our hands fell apart.

—

Every morning, I checked your bloodwork, paying particular attention to a graph of your bilirubin levels. After a couple of weeks, there was a significant steep descent back toward normal. I liked to imagine these levels as a countdown to you getting out of the hospital and getting your life — not just your labs — back toward normal.

By this time, I was trending toward a new normal myself. I now had *some* idea of what was going on: I knew my way around the hospital and no longer felt like fainting on rounds. I became more comfortable in my routine. You settled into a routine, too.

I remember on a particularly busy morning, I rushed through a physical exam.

"Doc," you reminded me, "Aren't you gonna check my lungs?"

I had become too comfortable.

I checked your lungs, embarrassed that I had forgotten such a crucial part of the exam. I was comforted by your familiar breaths, calmly and reliably cycling in and out.

"No changes," I reassured — though more for me than you.

"I got your back, buddy," you winked.

The only thing that seemed to change was your daily visitors. Usually your daughter. Your ex-wife and her new husband. Your brother. Your son. Your friend from the casino. Every day, in between other patients, lectures, meetings and other academic obligations, I'd say hello, meet a new friend or family member, and chat, catching scant slivers of who you were outside of the hospital.

At the end of each day, I'd check in on you.

"Get out of here, they're working you too hard," you'd say. I would see you the next day, and we'd start all over again. One day at a time.

—

There were good days: your new room, your procedure, your grandchildren. There were bad days: your fall, your diagnosis, your prognosis. On my last day, I had to finish an assignment, which involved interviewing you. You didn't want to talk at first, but once you started, I watched as you played clips from the past in your head, like you were showing me reels of your home movies in tones of sepia and amber: joining the Army, working after the war, watching football with your family.

I watched as you changed the reels, projecting crisp clips of your future: vacations you'd take once you were better, celebrations you'd be a part of, dreams of what you would do with more time.

I tucked my assignment away and just sat, hoping to one day hear that these dreams had become memories.

When I got up to leave, I reminded you it was my last day. You offered your hand and said, "Goodbye, buddy, I love ya." We shook hands, and I felt your rough palms, warm, honest, against mine.

I sat in my car and watched as the sun, tired after a long day, began its descent toward the horizon. As it declined, it turned the sky a stunning pastiche of orange, then pink, and then — just as it lay its head down for a well-deserved rest — it let out one last gasp of brilliant yellow before succumbing to the dark blue of night.

INTIMATE REFLECTIONS

Restrained
March 16, 2020

Madeline Fryer
University of Massachusetts Medical School
Class of 2021

I PROPOSED A DEAL TO my fellow student on our surgery rotation: "You can have all the other cases today if I get the laryngectomy."

"Sure," he sighed apathetically. "Whatever you want."

A total laryngectomy involves dissecting through the thyroid gland and small muscles of the neck to expose a person's airway. Intricate blood vessels and elusive nerve fibers are navigated to obtain a clean view, and then the connection from the patient's mouth to their windpipe, including their vocal cords, is removed. A new hole is created in the front of the patient's neck that allows air to reach their lungs. Important nerves that affect a person's ability to smile, move their tongue, shrug their shoulders, turn their head and take a deep breath are all at risk. At the end of the case, patients are left unable to speak.

This surgery is usually performed to treat an aggressive cancer, and it is always high-stakes. Laryngectomies are rare at my training hospital, and I did not want to miss the opportunity to participate.

My eager feet bolted down the stairs towards the pre-operative area, galloping in asynchronous parallel with my racing mind. I strained to remember textbook images I had reviewed the night before, knowing the anatomy would be much more disorienting in the flesh than in glossy labeled pages.

I restrained my eagerness as I introduced myself to the patient for the first time. It would be callous and insensitive to show such genuine excitement for a procedure that was about to render her permanently mute. She was more weatherworn than I expected; her withered frame was easily overlooked beneath the stack of impersonal hospital blankets specially engineered to shed fewer fibers. Her raspy greeting was barely audible over the maelstrom of surrounding nurses, patients and alarming monitors. I wondered if she used as few words as possible out of shyness, physical pain, or if she was already trying to prepare for life after her surgery.

When we finally arrived in the operating room, our patient tightly shut her eyes after one glance at the carefully arranged surgical instruments that would take away her organic voice. A heaviness nestled deep in my diaphragm that made each breath feel more drawn out and deliberate. The permanence of what we were about to inflict on this scared woman was oppressive and inescapable. I felt guilty wondering if the surgery I was so eager to be a part of would feel worthwhile to her in the end.

I took extra care in helping to position the patient on the table and explained every step before touching her: "These wraps will massage your legs and help prevent blood clots. I'm going to put them around your calves now." She silently nodded, and I wrapped them twice around her child-sized limbs.

"These foam pads will protect your heels from developing sores." Another nod, smaller this time.

"I'm going to place this belt around your waist to protect you from falling." This time she opened her eyes with a look that wondered if I was crazy, but she nodded a third time.

Per hospital protocol, the full OR team reviewed our patient's information and imminent procedure before the anesthesiologist put her to sleep. Sallow, heavy lids shielded her gaze from the harsh lights above, but tears rolling down her cheek betrayed the otherwise stoic demeanor lying supine on the table. The anesthesiologist dammed her silent weeping with sedative medication and two pieces of tape.

Twenty-five minutes later, my guilt ebbed away as I watched the attending and resident dissect down, plane after plane, identifying anatomy in views I had only seen in pictures. I reveled in the novelty of it all. I was having fun. There was no conscious patient for whom I needed to reign in my excitement; I was in the company of surgeons.

Jubilant violins and soulful folk singers warbled over the speakers to soundtrack our work. I felt the internal crescendo of each pulsating artery and elusive nerve safely dissected out of harm's way. I no longer noticed my own breathing or any other feeling in my body; it was as if I was hovering a few inches off the ground, weightless and unrestrained. I felt personally lighter with every lymph node and tissue section removed from the patient's throat.

After the incisions surrounding our patient's delicate new airway were coated with bacitracin, everyone in the room broke away for their respective jobs. The attending took his music and left to call her far-away family. Over the drone of the room's ventilation, the resident clacked away on a keyboard in the corner to write the operative note. The nurses were at the back table double-checking their instruments to ensure nothing was left behind, while the anesthesiologist read monitors and titrated gases. For a few moments, I was the only person to just stand and be with our patient. I watched her chest rise and fall in the midst of activity that was entirely about yet did not involve her at all.

As she began waking from anesthesia, I instinctively reached down and held her forearms to the bed as her hands started to reach up. Patients regaining consciousness can inadvertently injure their eyes and dislodge breathing tubes and IVs, and I didn't want anything unexpected to happen on my watch. As I pinned her arms to the bed, fear-filled hazel eyes pleaded with mine as I used increasing force to keep her arms down.

"Your surgery is all done. It went really well. You're still waking up in the operating room. Just rest your arms down!" I commanded her, hoping she would stop fighting me.

Tentatively she tried to speak but had been rendered completely mute by our scalpel. The only sound she could make was a soft pucker from her parting lips. I fumbled through an attempt at lip reading that frustrated us both. She gave up trying to speak and instead of lifting her arms up, she pushed them out to the side. I decided to let go, but she reached out and took my hand between hers. She smiled at me as I finally understood the word I failed to make out moments before: hand. I had been restraining a defenseless, frightened woman from trying to hold my hand.

In my overzealous effort to protect this woman from herself, I lost sight of what was happening in front of me. A vulnerable person who trusted us felt scared and alone, and she needed to be shown that we would be there for her and she would be alright. I moved so blindly through the motions of doing my job that I failed to recognize the most basic need for human connection.

We inflicted massive, irreversible damage to remove a tumor that might kill her anyway. Did we miss the mark there, too, in our enthusiasm to do good? This woman was counseled extensively about her treatment options, but it is difficult to ignore even the quietest whispers of guilt and self-doubt. There is often no clear answer for when the most aggressive treatment is the best one, and I worry that my excitement for innovative procedures will obscure what future patients need most. I might not get it right every time, but I will strive to be worthy of their trust, listen to what they tell me and help them wake up by holding their hands.

IN-TRAINING: 2020 IN OUR WORDS

Grief Unanswered
October 22, 2020

Sharon Hsu
Albany Medical College
Class of 2022

We sit in a makeshift ring
under fluorescent lights,
halfway into the allotted one hour
before we realize that we are having
a conversation born a decade ago.

He leads us to the day he died
and began again, unwillingly
made wise to the depth that the scalpel may cut —
through the skin and muscles
of his second youngest daughter,
all the way into his own heart.
To describe the gash it left
as a remnant is too forgiving; he bleeds,
unhealed.

"I will lose no more,"
he interrupts and cries,
silencing the translator
without imprint
on the urges of the doctors.
The third time he repeats himself,
his face is dry,
and still,
and cold —
"no more."

Outside the door,
we turn right
as he turns left,
and the projection of his weeping soul
lingers in the room
to play out the allotted one hour.

No surgery is scheduled
for the little boy down the hall
who crouches over a toy car
and runs it over bumps in the carpet,
waiting for his father.

IN-TRAINING: 2020 IN OUR WORDS

"I Can't Be Here Anymore"
September 26, 2020

Vidiya Sathananthan
East Tennessee State University Quillen College of Medicine
Class of 2021

IT WAS MY FIRST DAY back in the hospital since the COVID-19 pandemic began. Because of the long hiatus, I felt like a brand new third-year, lost and struggling to get a handle on the medicine service. During rounds, I was scrambling just to write notes and learn all the patients, but I paused when I saw Mr. K. He was in his 30s — not much older than I — but his skin clung to his bones, and his pallid face seemed hollow. The darkness under his eyes gave the impression of a fatigue that belied his years.

Mr. K had been admitted with dehydration and malnutrition secondary to diarrhea in the setting of HIV. During his stay, he developed refeeding syndrome. When the resulting electrolyte imbalances paved the way for cardiac arrhythmias, he coded twice in the ICU. The care team managed to bring him back each time but not without consequence: the brutality of numerous cycles of CPR left him with multiple rib fractures, inflicting sharp pain with every breath.

Two days after his last code, I tapped on the glass door of his ICU room during pre-rounds. He was watching the sun start to come up over the mountains into what was still a dark blue sky. He looked so small in that vast ICU room, taking up less space than all the equipment he was attached to.

I approached the edge of his bed and told him that his electrolyte levels were still too low for us to move him out of the ICU. Tears quickly filled his sunken eyes. He buried his face in his hands.

"I can't be here anymore. I need to leave. I will leave."

—

Over the next few days, our care team spent more time by Mr. K's bedside than with any other patient, exploring his desire to leave against medical advice (AMA). His discomfort and determination to leave only grew though. Each time I saw him, the weight of his anxiety was more and more apparent in the dark circles under his eyes, in the way he stared into the void of his empty room.

As his anxiety was intensifying, my team's patience was waning. The residents, already worn ragged by the toll of COVID-19, were tired of pleading with Mr. K to stay at least another 24 hours under our care, tired of explaining the severity of his illness, tired of reiterating why it was so dangerous for him to leave the safety of the ICU.

As clinicians, we become frustrated when our patients want to leave AMA. We cannot fathom why a patient would not want to take care of themselves or at least allow us to take care of them. Our tendency is to focus on educating the patient of the severity of their illness and the necessity of treatment. As with Mr. K, though, many of these patients fully understand their illness process and the need for hospitalization. We are sometimes unable to step back from the intricacies of adjusting electrolyte disturbances or after the stress of running a code to recognize that a patient is suffering from something we are not addressing.

When I think of Mr. K and of many of the other patients I've seen leave AMA, I can recognize the fear. I can recognize the dire loneliness that only comes from severe illness. It is the unique anxiety that comes from being sick and isolated in the hospital, away from both the comforts and constants of life outside of the hospital.

This anxiety is highly visible in COVID-19 patients. In fact, it has become recognized as part of COVID-19 care recommendations that this anxiety must be addressed to support the patient and improve their care.[1] However, despite multiple studies showing the value in addressing the psychological needs of patients with other conditions, we do not regularly extend this support to our general hospitalized population.[2] The consequences of not doing so can include increased risk of mortality, physical disability, post-traumatic stress disorder, or the decision to leave AMA and not continue with any treatment.

—

Late that week, I headed to Mr. K's room to attend a meeting regarding his treatment plan. When I walked in the door, I was taken aback by a transformation. His parents sat in chairs next to his bedside, and, with their arrival, the whole atmosphere had changed.

The cold cell of an ICU room now radiated the warmth and comfort of a room pictured in *Southern Living* magazine. Mr. K lounged against pillows from home on a bed covered with patchwork quilts. He still looked exhausted, but there was a light in his eyes now as the attending began the discussion.

"Your electrolyte levels continue to dip despite our efforts to replace them and give you appropriate nutrition. You're still not ready to leave the ICU."

Mr. K looked at his mother and simply shook his head with grief, his eyes too tired to fill with tears. Our team expected him to demand to leave again, perhaps with the support of his parents. At this point, Mr. K could easily articulate how his deficits in magnesium, potassium, and phosphate could cause another electrical abnormality in his heart and lead to death, but this knowledge didn't seem enough to overcome the anxiety he experienced stuck in the ICU. Our team watched in silence, waiting for Mr. K's refusal, but instead we heard something else.

"Son, I know it is hard being here. I hate that we can't be here with you all the time. But please don't leave. I watched them beat on your chest to keep you alive, and I can't bear for you to go through that again."

Mr. K's father had always been a quiet figure in the room each time he visited. His emotional plea was raw and heavy, but it came from a place of boundless love for his son. With it came Mr. K's willingness to stay in the ICU. Each day after that he appeared stronger, more resilient, bolstered by the support of his parents and the therapeutic alliance with his care team.

Though Mr. K did not have COVID-19, the emotional distress of his severe illness and the isolation were similar. As a medical student learning during this pandemic, I'm continually asking myself what I will take away from this strange and haunting period. With the backdrop of the global isolation we have all felt to an extent during this year, the ups and downs of Mr. K's journey highlight the need to be more intentional about assessing the psychosocial needs of any hospitalized patient — COVID-19 or not — especially in light of the new restrictions on family visiting. Though we must provide diagnostic and therapeutic care, we must also be vigilant about recognizing emotional distress in our patients and think creatively about how to address it.

Emptied
March 25, 2020

Rma Kumra
University of Nevada Reno School of Medicine
Class of 2020

THE ELECTRIC DOORS OPENED: Zo and I walked through the passageway to the PACU. Even at 12:30 a.m. the hallway was lined with people in purple scrubs: nurses, CNAs, and whoever else was staffed at this time. Chatter filled the usually quiet PACU. No beeping. Just the light conversation of night shift. Any time the electric doors opened, there would be silence. "False alarm!" someone would yell, and the chatter would resume.

The electric doors opened again, but this time no one yelled.

A hospital bed rolled in. It was Marvin. His last walk. On rounds we would say, "Twenty-two-year-old with GSW (gunshot wound) to the head. Waiting for organ donation." In the real world, that meant that Marvin had died by suicide. He had succeeded, but only kind of. He was brought in functionally brain-dead, but we had to wait for his brain to herniate to officially pronounce it. His organ donor status meant that we kept him alive until transplant. Finally, after a week of laying in the critical care unit waiting for organ harvest, he was here in the PACU.

Behind his bed, pushed by a nurse, was his family. Ten people. His mother was beside herself. The child she had raised, for whom she had weaved dreams of a wonderful life and who she had protected from the world, was leaving her empty-handed. As his family followed him to the door, their devastation was on display. No longer could they hide behind the curtain of his room or in the comfort of their home. There was nothing else they could do.

Tears filled the eyes of the bystanders. Empathy flowed freely in an area where nurses and doctors usually remained composed. Once the bed made it to the operating room door, each family member said their final goodbye. Marvin's grandmother leaned over to kiss him. They were handing him over to the doctors and nurses — the vultures waiting for his organs to save another human life. Somehow, it still didn't seem fair.

In the cold OR, I stood quietly hugging myself. The transplant surgeons stood at both sides of Marvin with the anesthesiologist at his head. For the first time since I began my surgery rotation I knew for certain the patient wouldn't leave the OR alive. Bryan, the transplant nurse and the orchestrator of this whole ordeal, asked for a pause. The eulogy started. This time I couldn't hold my tears back. Suddenly, the 22-year-old with a GSW became a whole human — loving rock-and-roll, playing with his pets, and seemingly happy — rather than fragments on a piece of paper. But there wasn't much time to linger on my emotions at the loss of a patient and a human being. It was time for the harvest.

Zo and I made our way to the head of the bed where I stood on a stool to get a better view of the operation. I witnessed the longest incision I had ever seen. He was exposed, his heart and his abdomen just splayed apart. The medical student in me was in awe. The beating heart trembled in the surgeon's hands: ventricular fibrillation. Over the next half hour, they continued to work on taking the heart out of his body.

Marvin remained alive. His brain had not been functional for a week now, but its remnants lay well hidden under the dressings over his head. Finally, the nurse introduced the infusion that would arrest Marvin's heart. His blood pressure plummeted. Marvin was gone, and there was no time to waste or grieve. The heart now belonged to a 42-year-old man a couple states away.

Measurements and packaging of the heart finished quickly, and the cardiology transplant team left. The GI team continued to take out the liver and kidneys. Part of me felt exhilarated to see this miracle of medicine, but another part of me just wanted to pause and grapple with the loss of someone I had never spoken to. Finally, only the OR staff was left. We helped them put Marvin in a body bag for a forensic pathologist to examine; he was empty. I thought about his family, how empty they must feel without him.

At 4:45 a.m., we finally walked out of the OR. Placed on the outside of the door was his high school graduation picture. Both Zo and I stared at it. Marvin seemed so innocent and happy, but who knew the chaos that had stirred inside his soul. Silently, we walked through the halls to the call room. Despite the near 24-hour shift, I didn't feel exhausted. All I felt was empty.

Marvin was my first patient to die and, in his death, he touched me in an inexplicable way. Maybe it was the loss of a life that could have been, maybe it was that I related to his struggle with mental illness, or maybe it was the inconsolable grief of a family. I'm still not quite sure. However, what I do know is that I will never forget him and that feeling: empty.

INTIMATE REFLECTIONS

The Infinite
April 9, 2020

Meagan Campbell
University of Minnesota Medical School
Class of 2023

Blue latex feels slick against
my hands. I grip my instrument tightly,
surprised breath escaping me as
the scalpel quickly reveals
glistening unknown beneath.
As we work in tandem to expose the
knowledge we seek, I ponder what memories
this body has known.

While my hands slice and reveal, I see
vibrant sunsets, earth-shattering heartbreaks,
Sundays at the park.
I imagine dreary workdays,
passionate embraces, rain-soaked windows,
every shimmering facet once contained in this
chrysalis before me.

I will never know each faded childhood memory,
the favorite crisp linen shirt, every midnight kiss.
We are ephemeral beings,
brilliant and glittering for only an instant.
Yet within this speck of light
is unconditional love, laughter, and hazy afternoon baseball games.
Within each pearly dewdrop is contained
the infinite.

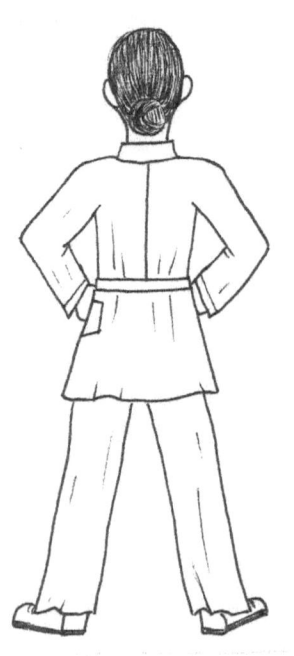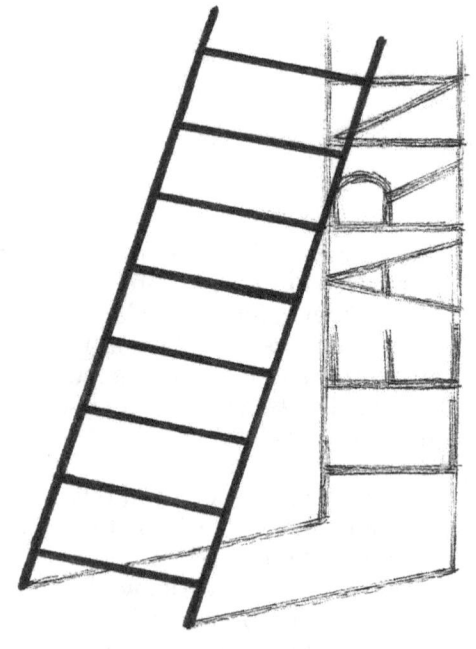

Reimagining #MedEd

•

culture

Yes, Doctor

June 29, 2020

Rohan Patel
American University of the Caribbean School of Medicine
Class of 2020

YES, DOCTOR.
I am running through the fluorescent-lit halls in my short white coat, pockets full of God knows what — surgical lubricant, suturing kits, saline flushes, pens and mystery stains from the day prior. Catching up to the group, I fall in line as we gather to begin rounds. I prepare to answer any question on the patient's prognosis. Instead, my attending glares at me intently and asks for scissors. No amount of caffeine in my veins can erase my blank look as I stare back at the surgeon. *I prepared for everything and still forgot the scissors.* I scramble, sifting through my pockets for anything to help, but he has already written me off to discuss medications with a resident.

Two years of intense studying should have culminated in a feeling of strength. I ended my second year of medical school thinking I was now prepared to do anything. I was excited to be a problem-solver, armed with the mental acuity to recognize diseases from A to Z, ready to proceed with the next step in my clinical training. Now, in my third year, it is finally time to act like a *real* doctor. But our superiors treat us like their personal assistants.

Yes, doctor, I will run down these blood samples while you finish the procedure.

Yes, I'd be happy to bother the radiologist a third time to read the scan immediately.

Yes, I can definitely grab some coffee for you.

We listen carefully and execute tasks precisely, yet this still feels wrong. Why is it that all we can do is be "yes men" to senior doctors? Why aren't we treated like the professionals we are training so diligently to become?

As we exit the room of our last postoperative patient, a shared sense of comfort settles among the students. We survived the chopping block, but now the next phase begins. As the rounding team disassembles, we rush to review the charts of our assigned cases. As if sprinting in a race, we pore over every minute detail, every comorbidity, every previous note we can read in five minutes. With an air of confidence, I head off to introduce myself to my next patient in the preoperative holding area.

Everything is in order as the attending and resident walk in to speak with the patient. The stern surgeon reviews the upcoming surgery with the patient: a simple laparoscopic removal of fibroids in the woman's uterus. Trailing behind quietly, I mentally go over the possible questions I could be asked during the procedure. Just as I get lost in my thoughts, I bump into the surgeon.

He turns around and asks me point blank, "Can you do me a favor? The patient doesn't have any family members picking her up after the surgery. I will pay for your Uber to drop her off home and return to the hospital." I blink, perplexed and thrown off by such an unusual request. I look at my resident for guidance, but she purposely avoids eye contact.

"Yes, doctor," I smile, "Just give me her address and the time I should take her home."

Determined to make an impression, I have become the "yes man" I so despise. My attending's eyes light up as he promises to reward me upon my return. My resident knows all too well the position I am in but leaves for the OR without a word.

My worries over the liability of taking a patient home, the risk of going off on my own and the surgeon's disappointment in my abilities grow throughout the day. Uncomfortable with this task, I weigh the potential consequences of my options. As I vent to my classmates over lunch, the chief resident pulls me aside. She reassures me that a decision to deny my attending's request will not reflect poorly on my evaluation. She will speak with the attending to find alternative means for the patient to get home safely.

Relief starts to settle over me, but the unnerving feeling that I had crossed an unforgiving boundary lingers longer than expected. Like rungs on a ladder, the hierarchy of the medical profession places experienced physicians at the top and medical students at the very bottom. How can we speak out when our seniors loom so high overhead?

From the beginning, we are taught to be "team players" with the underlying expectation that we should always be ready to assist no matter the circumstances. But it does not take long for us to realize that when we do not meet our superior's expectations, no matter how unrealistic, we are deemed unworthy of our superior's energy or attention.

Are our voices so small that we need to keep quiet, even when it goes against our morals? Have we abandoned our goal of becoming physicians only to become our seniors' assistants? Are we ungrateful for not wanting to listen to the teachers who are training us to be better physicians? Is our worth defined by one small mistake? Are we only deserving of one chance?

No, doctor.

As I continue to mull over the daunting repercussions of defying my attending, the chief resident winks at me as she heads to the OR in my stead. "Rohan, enjoy your day," she says. She smiles and fearlessly walks off, giving me confidence that everything will be alright. Like my guardian angel, my resident had come to my aid, showing me that I don't have to fight this battle alone.

That day, I learned a valuable lesson. When we as medical students graduate into the long white coat, we must realize that we will inevitably impact the next generation of doctors. Mistreatment and disrespect should not be a culture that we perpetuate or that our juniors become accustomed to. The practice of collaboration can easily overpower the hierarchical negativity that some doctors spread. Like the chief resident who defended my position to the stern attending, we must reclaim the phrase "*yes, doctor.*"

By validating our struggles while advocating for our juniors, we can set the tone that respect is the new norm. After all, we must encourage growth and empower our colleagues to be their best selves. We must realize the gravity of our roles and treat peers and colleagues accordingly. Within a new culture that fosters empowerment, it will be easy for us to come together and proudly say, *yes, doctor.*

Welcome to Medicine
September 16, 2020

Apshara Ravichandran
Saint Louis University School of Medicine
Class of 2022

YOU DON'T DESERVE abuse because you're a medical student. You don't have to "take it" because you're a medical student.

You don't have to sit in silence and painfully nod along with an attending's racist, misogynist lectures because you're their medical student. You don't need to pick the skin off your cuticles to stop yourself from replying. You don't need to learn how to hide your grimaces behind your mask because you know you'll have to listen to them attack your identity for the next several weeks.

My first interaction with my new attending immediately set off alarm bells in my head: when I introduced myself, he commented on what a difficult name I had and asked twice if he could call me "Abby." Throughout the day, he would go on to flippantly joke about mental illness and homicide, spread false beliefs about COVD-19, refuse to wear a mask in patient rooms and call every female in the office (including patients as well as myself) inappropriate pet names. As he casually spouted countless racist or sexist views, I held my tongue and hid my discomfort. This rotation was 1:1 with the attending and without other medical students, interns, or residents to validate my concern, I convinced myself I would just have to make it through the next two months.

From just one day in the clinic, I had compiled a list of 13 bullet points that outlined the most obviously questionable comments and actions from my attending. But I still didn't trust my experience — was I overreacting? Was I being too sensitive? Was I going to ruin this attending's life by voicing my concerns? As "just a med student," did I even deserve the right to feel uncomfortable?

When I tentatively mentioned to friends the litany of offensive, problematic statements my attending physician had said during the first two days of my rotation, a common response was, "Welcome to medicine." That struck a nerve. I didn't want to accept that statement as fact, I didn't want to accept this environment as inevitable and I didn't feel that we, as the next generation of physicians, should have to. More than my own discomfort, it was the frustrating complacency enveloped in "welcome to medicine" that finally convinced me to reach out to my school about the attending.

When I came forward, I realized that I had the most supportive medical school administration I could have hoped for. They made it clear that they were on my side from my very first tentative question: "Is this really that bad?" They took me seriously and removed me from that rotation the minute they heard my concerns. I felt like my safety was their only priority. and I'm grateful for that.

Even with this overwhelming support, I was hesitant to bring my concerns to my administration — and I wasn't alone in that uncertainty. The 2019 Graduation Questionnaire by the American Association of Medical Colleges (AAMC) noted that 40.1% of graduating medical students experienced mistreatment during their time in medical school; only 23.2% of those students reported their experience.[1] Students cited fear of retaliation, doubt that an event was important enough to report, and the belief that nothing would be done about the situation as reasons for not reporting.

These were all thoughts that ran through my head; at the bottom of the hierarchy of medical education, we don't trust ourselves enough to believe that what feels wrong might actually be wrong. Most insidiously, a 2018 study found that one of the leading reasons medical students don't report mistreatment during their clinical years is the perception that mistreatment is a normal part of medical education, a rite of passage if you will.[2]

"Welcome to medicine."

These statistics truly hit home for me after I left my rotation when I heard that the other attending physicians at the office were whispering about "that poor medical student" who "did the right thing" by leaving the placement. Those physicians discussed amongst themselves how that attending had become increasingly problematic and how schools shouldn't assign students to that person anymore. They had known before my name had ever even shown up in the office inbox that this attending was a questionable teacher and provider.

I struggled with pangs of betrayal and loneliness: these physicians had nodded to me in the hallways and had gossiped about "that poor medical student" in private. While I was fielding microaggressions one-on-one across a desk, berating myself to get a grip, fighting against my own instincts, they had known all along that I was going to struggle and left me to flounder anyway. Those white male physicians with the most power to protect students from an objectionable teacher did nothing. I don't know why they felt like they had to wait for a third-year medical student to speak out before they could, but I can't help but wonder: perhaps they, too, thought, "Welcome to medicine."

I didn't learn much medicine the first week of my rotation, but I learned something else: that I don't want to subscribe to the culture of medicine that makes students believe they have to tough it out. Medicine isn't an old boys' club anymore. No matter how low we may be in the medical hierarchy, we deserve respect. If we can't count on those in positions of power to advocate for us, then we will have to advocate for ourselves.

I don't mean to say that there aren't thoughtful, supportive attendings that continue to fight for us — there are, and I've had the privilege of working with many of them. This experience has shown me, however disappointing the thought may be, that I can't necessarily count on that. But the old guard is not the future of medicine — we are. And we can work towards a better system than "welcome to medicine."

IN-TRAINING: 2020 IN OUR WORDS

The Vulnerability of Our Patients and Ourselves: A Parallel Chart Reflection

October 6, 2020

Rachel Fields
Florida International University Herbert Wertheim College of Medicine
Class of 2021

I ACTUALLY DON'T REMEMBER his name; he wasn't my patient. I just saw him on rounds every day during my internal medicine clerkship. He was in his late 80s, and he was very ill. He had a long history of COPD, most likely attributed to his even longer history of smoking. He had been admitted to our service for a severe respiratory infection a few days prior to me starting the rotation. This was my last rotation of my third year, and I walked in thinking I had seen enough COPD patients to know exactly what to expect.

The first day I saw him, he was angry and frustrated. He was alert and annoyed as the attending, three residents and three medical students filed into his room. All of us students stood there quietly, totally useless, staring at him like a zoo animal while the attending offered few words with little meaning behind them. Something along the lines of "we're doing everything we can" or "you're getting the best possible care." He finished the encounter with "so, we'll see what happens," which I later learned was the attending's default response when he didn't have a definitive answer for his patients.

I don't remember much else about this first encounter, but I clearly recall the attending's reaction when we left the room: "It's his fault he's this sick; he still is smoking every day. It's his fault he requires so much oxygen and is having such a poor response to the infection. He is self-destructive and killing his lungs."

I have heard physicians and students say things to this effect so many times at this point, and it still makes me immensely uncomfortable every time. Usually, it's a morbidly obese patient admitted for shortness of breath, or a drug addict admitted for withdrawal. Regardless, I instantly feel for the patient — and just moments later I feel weak and ashamed for being affected by these patients and their stories. I feel a desire to protect and defend these patients. Of course, I am not brave enough (or reckless enough, maybe) to stand up to an attending physician and counter his thoughts and opinions as he blames these patients for their shortcomings.

Why do I feel differently from these physicians who can look past the vulnerability of these patients? Is it good or bad that I am affected by these patients and their tragedies? Does it make me weak or does it make me understanding and compassionate? And then I feel a whole new level of shame for even having these thoughts. Of course it's okay to feel and connect with my patients! The thought of becoming jaded or ambivalent towards my patients terrifies me even more than being considered an overly emotional physician.

Either way, at that moment, standing there listening to the attending pass judgment on the man's choices, I was sympathetic toward his suffering. Whether or not his condition was self-inflicted, the patient was old, sick, alone, exhausted and giving up — and I thought that deserved some compassion.

It was easy the first few days to see this patient. He was out of breath, pale and a little diaphoretic but otherwise "normal." His irritability was his most observable symptom in those first few days. He was relatively nice and polite when I talked to him, but I could tell he was exhausted and discouraged, and it was causing him to be easily agitated. But as his condition worsened and his body deteriorated, his entire presentation changed.

He was the first patient I had ever seen who sounded like he was literally drowning in his own respiratory secretions. The gurgling noise of someone fighting to breathe with every inhale and exhale was a scary noise that stayed with me long after leaving the patient's room. It was enough to churn my stomach and make my heart race at the very real promise of eventual respiratory failure.

As the patient's respiratory symptoms continued to progress and his health further deteriorated, one attending finished his week and the next attending began. The incoming attending demonstrated a softer approach, and I felt more at ease as he spoke about his patients. His words were kinder. He took more time and gathered more of the patient's story. His words and actions were tender, and his compassion for the patient built a more intimate connection in one day than the other attending seemed to build in an entire week.

He was older than the other attending and maybe a little wiser — or maybe just a little more empathetic. I found comfort in his approach as I could tell this patient was likely going to be transitioned to comfort measures as the next step in his plan of care.

As a medical student, I often find myself standing in the background while the attendings and residents talk to the patients during rounds. During pre-rounds, I try to demonstrate some confidence and authority with "my" patients and act sure in my role as their student-physician. However, during rounds, as the low person on the totem pole, I find myself often relying on body language to give any meaning to my presence in the room. I try to make eye contact and give a polite nod or encouraging smile. Sometimes it's a little awkward, but those few motions are my attempt at giving myself purpose in order to feel less out of place.

On the last day I saw this patient, he was hooked up to BiPAP and was only capable of nodding and moving his hands because any form of talking or other activity required too much exertion, and he did not possess the stamina. Feeling embarrassed and impudent, I gave an awkward wave to the patient. He returned my gesture, and my heart sank. He looked so vulnerable and exhausted raising his thin, bony fingers to reciprocate.

It was a pitiful sight, really, seeing a grown man like that. Seeing someone so ill that he can't walk or talk or use the bathroom but still has the mental capacity to know what others must see when looking at him. I felt like an intruder on a private and demeaning experience as this patient lost his dignity with each labored breath.

The vulnerability of grown men and women during illness is something I was unprepared for when starting medical school. I can't help to think that so many of our patients must feel so naked and exposed as they lay in their beds in their various stages of sickness and health as we flow in and out of their rooms in our clean white coats, professional attire, brushed hair and make-up. How helpless this must make them feel. In recognizing these feelings of helplessness and weakness, I too often feel defenseless, exposed and embarrassed as well.

The patient died sometime over the next few days. I'm not sure exactly how events unfolded as the medical students did not round with the team over the weekend. But on Monday when I asked the resident where this man was, he looked in the chart and saw he had been discharged, readmitted and eventually succumbed to his illness in the ED.

I felt this was a tragic end to a tragic story. He did not die in his home or surrounded by family; he did not even die in the comfort of a private hospital room. He died between two curtains in the chaotic, overcrowded ED. When this information was shared with me I took a breath, prayed a silent prayer and returned to work with my team hoping that my little prayer was not the only moment through which this patient would be mourned and remembered.

Becoming More Emotionally Intelligent, Adaptive Physician-Leaders

December 26, 2020

Ashten Duncan
OU-TU School of Community Medicine
Class of 2021

THE COVID-19 PANDEMIC has taken the world by storm, causing upheavals in every area of life. Given the need to follow social distancing and other infectious disease prevention guidelines, physicians and other health care professionals have had to adjust their approaches to providing care.[1,2] Depending on the setting in which they work, more physicians have been using telehealth and telemedicine platforms like Doximity and Amwell to conduct patient visits without crowding their waiting rooms.[3]

As part of the Coronavirus Aid, Relief, and Economic Security (CARES) Act, the Centers for Medicare and Medicaid Services (CMS) enacted a policy for telehealth payment parity.[4,5] This policy change has enabled many physicians and other providers working in largely outpatient practices to stay afloat during this tumultuous time. However, many practices continue to struggle despite this accommodation.[6]

For those of us training and working in health care, it is a foregone conclusion that changes in health care practices are inevitable and often occur at full pelt. As a fourth-year medical student, I have been straddling the line between undergraduate medical education and supervised residency training. This has given me a unique view of the multitudes of adjustments that programs have made in the wake of both the Liaison Committee on Medical Education (LCME) and Accreditation Council for Graduate Medical Education (ACGME) recommendations.[7,8] While many United States-based medical training programs have resumed mostly normal clinical rotation schedules, there remains enduring modifications, including a greater emphasis on telehealth training and appropriate prioritization of non-emergent care.[9,10]

All of these abrupt paradigm shifts have left patients and providers alike scrambling to plan out procedures, routine health maintenance visits and screenings.[11] With the Pfizer, Moderna and other prominent COVID-19 vaccine candidates proceeding rapidly through Phase 3 clinical trials and now being rolled out en masse, many are wondering what next year will be like for daily life.[12]

Sadly, the general population continues to be subjected to the inexorable spread of misinformation and disinformation with no equal in the history of our country.[13] Effectively, physicians have become the front-line infantry in the war on science.[14] While there are numerous reasons for the cultural shift toward distrusting science as an institution, the fact remains that physicians have to pick up the mantle and defend the paramountcy of rigorous scientific inquiry.

For several decades, the role of the physician has evolved from the traditional diagnostician, preventer and treater of human disease described in the biomedical model into a more integrated "biopsychosocial" practitioner.[15,16] Current evidence suggests that much of human health is influenced more significantly by contextual factors like the social determinants of health than the direct receipt of health care.[17] This relatively new understanding has challenged the notion of "physicianhood" and what it means to improve the health of entire populations and communities.[18] With the influx of issues that the pandemic has brought with it, this new model for being a highly effective physician has become even more important.

Studies have demonstrated that skeptics of evidence-based recommendations will still trust their physician's word on the importance of following those recommendations.[19] For example, clinical research has demonstrated that patients who have strong relationships with their primary care providers are more likely to adopt challenging health behaviors, such as taking medications as prescribed.[20] Additionally, adequate messaging around public health matters and health policy changes requires the input of physicians who have been in the trenches and can advocate compellingly for their communities' needs.[21]

For us to be successful, physicians have to be in tune with their creativity and adaptive leadership skillset.[22] These adaptive leadership skills include emotional intelligence, organizational justice, development and character. The days of operating as a lone wolf without much oversight are long gone; we have to accept that we are irrevocably in a time of increasing integration. Although one could lament the loss of individual autonomy as a practitioner, I would argue that this age brings with it a wealth of opportunity for professional growth and innovation.

One of the most important areas for innovation lies in cultivating a greater capacity for emotional intelligence in our health care workforce.[23] In the 1990s, Peter Salovey and John Mayer described the concept of emotional intelligence and how it was a cultivable trait involved in the awareness of and application of observed emotions to oneself and others.[24] Well known for his work in this area, Daniel Goleman built on this body of work by introducing the foundational concepts of emotional intelligence: 1) self-awareness, 2) self-management, 3) social awareness and 4) social skills.[25]

Since then, robust evidence has demonstrated how emotional intelligence can be developed and how it matters more than past achievement or classical intelligence in many cases.[26,27] As outlined in their book Leadership 2.0, Travis Bradberry and Jean Greaves show how emotional intelligence is the cornerstone of adaptive leadership, which enables excellence in leadership above and beyond the core leadership skillset.[28]

What makes emotional intelligence so critical as the concept of "physicianhood" changes is that this psychosocial quality allows physicians to flourish in the vicissitudes of turbulent times, such as this raging pandemic.[29] For example, one study of nurses showed how emotional intelligence moderates the stress-burnout relationship, implicitly serving as a potential resilience factor for those working in health care.[30]

Moreover, the qualities of the highly emotionally intelligent — and, per the late Stephen Covey, highly effective — person provide the necessary skills to work through and address the intense underlying fears and vexation of people who reject modern science and medicine.[31] While it can be easy to look at their arguments and either dismiss them or become irate by them, it is imperative that we understand that everyone wants to live a good, happy and healthy life. This means we must develop as professionals and become more capable of tackling the issues that the recent social and political environment has precipitated.[32]

What this year has made clear is that physicians must grow in areas previously underemphasized in medical training. To take on the challenge of online echo chambers casting aspersions on health professionals and the underlying fear many people have about what it takes to have good health, we need emotionally intelligent, adaptive physician-leaders.[33] We have role models whose examples we should emulate all across our country. This skillset extends far beyond what the borderline pejorative "soft skill" might imply and likely will matter much more than our technical knowledge in restoring faith in and support of the foundation on which the house of medicine is built.

Reimagining #MedEd

•

wellness

Medical Students Do Not Owe You Their Trauma

July 1, 2020

Tabitha Moses
Wayne State University School of Medicine
MD-PhD Trainee

IN THE MIDST OF multiple crises — the COVID-19 pandemic, the continued attacks on Black people and subsequent protests against police brutality, the removal of transgender health care rights and so much more — I have heard discussion about how these issues will be reflected in medical school, residency and related fields' interviews.[1-4] Specifically, it will become standard for interviewers to ask about how these events affected applicants, how they reacted to these events and whether they were personally impacted. On the surface, the inclination to ask these questions appears reasonable; however, this approach may actually be crass and devoid of any understanding on a personal level.

Interviewers who ask these questions in a professional setting typically consider these issues to be academic — purely topics for discussion that might provide useful insight into the way the applicant views the world. But for applicants who have been affected, these issues are not merely academic and their discussion can invoke significant emotional turmoil. So before we continue to tacitly accept this shift in interviewing, it is important to consider its purpose and impact on those being interviewed.

I remember only one of my medical school interviews clearly. The interviewer shook my hand, told me his name, gestured at me to sit down and before I had even fully taken my seat, asked, "So, how did your brother die?" I had written about my brother's death in a few of my essays where it seemed relevant — as a way to provide insight into my own experiences. In writing about it, I understood the implication that I consented to discuss the topic and, as such, I was able to answer his question with minimal hesitation. Nevertheless, the question itself and the way in which it was asked left me startled and uncomfortable with both the interviewer and the type of institution that would condone this interview style.

At the time, I interpreted the interviewer's approach as a tactic, a method of testing my ability to respond and stay composed under stressful, potentially upsetting situations. I had been warned that some schools trained interviewers to ask stressful questions with this purpose in mind. The school in question accepted me, so I will assume that I passed that test. Nonetheless, I think the test itself is wildly inappropriate and indicative of the type of destructive culture that some still find acceptable in medicine. This same culture allows faculty and physicians to ask students why they want to go into a field like psychiatry or addiction medicine with a certain look, one which betrays the fact that they are hoping for a particularly graphic answer.

In my situation, one could argue that I consented to discuss the topic by including it in an essay; therefore, no matter how the topic was broached, I was obligated to engage. But it is important to recognize that one disclosure does not automatically permit the recipient to probe deeper. In a case of a sexual assault, for example, the disclosure of having been assaulted does not give the listener permission to ask for details of the assault. For most, this example seems obvious, but, when extended to other potentially traumatic situations, the point appears to be lost.

Students who disclose their queer identity do not owe the listener details of how their family responded when they came out. Likewise, students who state that they spent their formative years in a war-torn country are not giving permission to be asked about the potential traumas they experienced while there.

The interviewer must consider the purpose of their questions and whether it is necessary to even broach certain topics. Some questions are asked either to "test" the applicant or satisfy the interviewer's curiosity, neither of which are appropriate motivations. In those few cases where there may be a meaningful reason to address trauma, questions should be respectful and should not seek more detail than has already been provided. Because, ultimately, the person sharing that vulnerable information should make the decision on what and how much they want to share. Regardless of the situation or the power dynamic, details are never owed.

The examples above are largely situations in which the person has some degree of choice in whether trauma is disclosed; however, there are people whose traumatic experiences are immediately seen without any form of consent. Race, gender and many disabilities are often visible and assumed. Consequently, those folks already know how quickly assumptions are made and the negative implications that can result. Although there are laws restricting certain questions in medical school and residency interviews — particularly as they relate to marginalized identities — these laws do not prevent more insidious questions and assumptions that can be even more personal and painful.[5]

While an interviewer cannot ask a student their ethnicity, for many students of color this is not something that can be hidden. Plus, interviewers are allowed to ask probing questions about how racism affects the applicant or even their thoughts on protests, such as those occurring now against police brutality. And, inevitably, when a Black student is asked about their thoughts on the current movement, it is not the same as when the question is asked to a White student. There is the unspoken "as a Black student…" that precedes the question and that forces the applicant to consider their own identity, community and traumas when responding.

For example, police violence is the leading cause of death for young Black Americans; the odds of a Black man dying at the hands of the police are 1 in 1,000.[6] This real and constant threat results in deep-rooted trauma and fear that many Black Americans as well as other minority groups have to experience every day.[7] So, forcing these distressing conversations onto vulnerable and already underrepresented students during an interview is unnecessary and, frankly, inhumane.

I recognize that interviews aim to gauge many aspects of applicants, including how they handle tough situations. But those questions can be answered without requiring students to re-experience and disclose traumas. Instead, ask applicants whether they have experienced difficulties with patients in clinics and how they handled them. That leaves the conversation open for the responder to also discuss more personal experiences if they feel comfortable doing so.

Ultimately, the legacy of medical training is rooted in the concept that students must be broken down and humiliated in order to learn effectively.[8-10] We are just now beginning to recognize that this is not the best way to train healthy physicians, and there have been wide-reaching efforts to change this system.[11,12] These changes must extend to the interview process. Interviews are fundamentally stressful, and there is an intrinsic power imbalance. We should not allow the use of this dynamic to force eager applicants to disclose issues and experiences that are inherently traumatizing. Because they do not owe you their trauma.

Do I Belong Here?
December 2, 2020

Rohan Patel
American University of Caribbean School of Medicine
Class of 2020

BECAUSE I'LL NEVER be good enough.
That creeping feeling that lurks in the back of your mind. Always present, but never too loud. It whispers in your ear, sowing seeds of doubt throughout every action.

Because they'll find out that I don't know anything.

I fight off this *noise* as I present my next patient during morning rounds. I dart my eyes up to seem like I am a robot reading word-for-word off my notes, focusing on my confidence while reciting my systems-based plan for my ICU patient.

Because I have one more mistake until I am exposed.

I am quickly interrupted by my attending. She asks me about the mechanism behind a dropping electrolyte level, and I respond with hesitation. Fortunately, my answer is exactly what she was looking for, and I continue on with my presentation. But that *noise* creeps back in my mind as the resident begins presenting the next patient.

The *noise* is the constant feeling of inadequacy and self-doubt. It manifests itself like a huge sea within the mind. Some days, you are just standing on the shore with the tides low and the waves calm. Other days, you are washed away in the middle of a storm, struggling to stay afloat, surrounded by waves hundreds of feet high. The deeper you are pulled into the dark abyss, the harder it is to swim to the surface. It pressures you to think that no matter how strong you are, you'll never overcome the strength of this force.

This phenomenon of *imposter syndrome* is prevalent in many of us pursuing medicine. Especially for those of us who are first-generation physicians, we are left to fend through uncharted territories. While we try to do our best to navigate this difficult path, we are left feeling that there is someone else better suited for our spot in medicine. We feel that we are not deserving of this privilege. As we pass through these high obstacles — basic sciences, board exams, core rotations, even electives — we stew in self-doubt after each success.

Because it was probably pure luck that I did well.

Feeling like some imposter overall takes a toll on our physical and mental health.[1] While our successes are displayed on paper, we can never celebrate it, let alone take credit for it. Such behaviors are key factors that lead to the ever-growing problem of physician burnout.[1] Due to burnout, more physicians are overwhelmed with emotional exhaustion, lack empathy and become cynical.

Because they are way smarter than I am.

We are constantly competing against our peers, regardless of the subtlety. Whether it is the class rank or getting the best evaluations in our rotations, this age of social clout puts undue burden on its participants. The exhaustion due to the juggling act of extracurriculars, research and licensing exams deprives us of the empathy and excitement that we once had when we first began our journey. This culture of competition roots itself deep in medicine and truly begins before the first day we step foot in the hospital or clinic, let alone a medical school classroom. The worst part of *imposter syndrome* is the idea that you are alone in exhibiting these emotions. But it is important to remember, you are never alone.

Because we are going to get through this together.

Don't let anyone tell you that they haven't experienced this before. You will always find someone who has doubts in their own abilities and accomplishments. It is realizing that your journeys are unique to you and cannot be compared equally amongst your peers. While you may think that they have everything figured out, you truly do not know what may actually be going on behind the scenes.

Because I am accomplished.

Reminding yourself of your successes is key. You were not given an acceptance to medical school by chance. You worked hard to pass through all the obstacles in your path, so celebrate it! Read through your old recommendation letters, read through your awards from year one, read through the essays you wrote at the height of your passion for medicine. Relish in the fact that you have come so far from where you first started. And remember to focus on self-love as you move up in the field, as that is the most infectious way to uplift ourselves and our community.

Because I am NOT an imposter.

A Defense of My Suicidal Peers
July 13, 2020

May Chammaa
Wayne State University School of Medicine
Class of 2022

Editor's note: We publish this article with a content warning due to discussions of suicide, suicidal ideation and depression.

—

A MEDICAL STUDENT, TO WHOM I will refer as X, posted on their social media page that they were going to kill themselves. Their letter was direct, raw and, as many suicide notes tend to be, apologetic. They explained they felt they no longer had the strength to keep fighting; it was simply "time for them to go."

The responses to this letter, as many responses to such notes tend to be, were well-intentioned but incongruent relative to the honest words in the original post. X confessed they were exhausted; people replied, "But we love you..." X painted a detailed and deliberate picture of internal suffering; people said, "But you're so handsome..." X said they were going to kill themselves; people answered, "We hope everything is okay." The next day, a friend updated everyone that X was doing "great" and reassured us that X is an outstanding person who enjoyed their life, felt bad about writing the suicide note and would never really kill themselves.

What strikes me in this situation is the stigmatized societal influence which results in feelings of guilt by the person who is already in a vulnerable position. Overwhelming and varying emotions after a suicide attempt are expected; however, I think guilt ought not to be part of this array. It is not my intent to encourage suicide or suicidal ideation; on the contrary, I write this with the aim of offering a defense for X and to contribute to destigmatizing the issue.

Being an outstanding person and wanting to die are not mutually exclusive. Sylvia Plath was terrified of what she described as a dark thing that sleeps in her; Elizabeth Wurtzel fell in love with her all-consuming depression because she felt it was all she had, all she was.[1,2] She described that she wished she could walk through a picture window and have the sharp broken shards slash her to ribbons so she could finally look how she felt.

Suicide should not be referred to as a terrible, abstract act that is shameful and unspeakable. Dr. Beth Brodsky, Associate Clinical Professor of Medical Psychology in Psychiatry at Columbia University, has commented on the high rate of physician suicide as "alarming" and affirmed that "suicide is an illness and not a crime."[3] There is a difference between discouraging someone from ending their life and making them feel guilty or ashamed of their feelings and actions, especially since this is not an uncommon occurrence.

According to the Centers for Disease Control, suicide was the second leading cause of death after unintentional injury for people between the ages of 10 to 34 in 2017.[4] This means suicide is a more common cause of death in this age group than homicide, malignant neoplasms, congenital abnormalities or heart disease. A majority of suicides and suicide attempts are associated with psychiatric disease, estimated to be at least 10 times higher risk than the general population.[5,6] Causes of suicide in the general population are extremely varied, including issues with finances, relationships, chronic disease diagnoses, discrimination, violence, terror and war.[6] Suicide is a tormenting and pertinent issue regardless of the specific etiology or risk factors.

Importantly, medical students have been reported to have higher rates of mental illness, burnout and depression than the general population; they are also less likely to receive treatment, with stigma as one of the barriers to treatment utilization. Thus, there is a need to reduce the stigma associated with mental illness.[7]

We must take care when trying to be supportive to avoid unintentionally perpetuating stigma and guilt. Referring to the well-established "but people love you" response is not effective; usually, suicidality is independent of a person's family, friends and peers. In fact, this response is more likely to externalize guilt and shame. Commenting on how "beautiful the person is" pointedly ignores their pain and is more likely to undervalue their feelings during a crisis. Posts expressing hopes that "everything is okay" when they are clearly not might be perceived as insensitive.

Regardless of the situation and your connection to a person like X, it is difficult and frightening to witness someone you care for in anguish. This fear may be the reason for a kind of paralysis of not finding the "right words" to say what you feel: I am here for you, and I want to help. While trying to express this caring sentiment, we ought to stay away from responses, well-intentioned as they may be, that allow stigma and guilt to flourish and solidify. Instead, aim to validate feelings, listen patiently and provide connections with community resources and treatment options.

If there is a need for urgent care, seeking help at an emergency department is appropriate. If you feel comfortable, remind them that you are there for them and ask how you can be supportive. In an ideal world, no one would feel compelled to post such a message on social media; I hope anyone in a similar situation feels able to reach out for guidance from trained specialists, using resources such as a suicide or crisis hotline, the American Psychiatric Association, the World Health Organization or the Suicide Prevention Resource Center.[8,9]

Lastly, dear X, I can only imagine how difficult it was for you to be vulnerable in front of your loved ones and peers. If you felt bad after the incident, I hope it was solely because of the nausea of the antidote, the IV in your arm, or maybe the hospital's uncomfortable pillows but not because of the burden of feeling that you need to apologize or redeem yourself. In a world filled with deception, your words were genuine and your choice to embrace help in the midst of your struggles was heartening and brave. I hope you are able to access the support you need to work through this, and I am excited to see the virtuous impact you will have on our communities and the medical field.

Soulful Medicine
September 21, 2020

Eric Bethea
Emory University School of Medicine
Class of 2022

TO MY SURPRISE, tears welled up in my eyes as the voice on the line said a soft prayer for my future success and safety. That voice belonged to Reverend Angela Johnson, former Spiritual Health Fellow and current provisional elder in the United Methodist Church; we were finishing up our discussion of the role of spirituality in medicine.

In that moment, I remember being touched at once by both the compassion required to call on a higher power for a stranger and by the comfort I received from the words themselves. At the time, I assumed that my tears were a product of being overcome by the sentiment of her words. Her prayers had been a final, heartfelt plea for me to take seriously the content of our conversation. Her earnestness could have softened even the staunchest skeptic.

However, after I had spent some time processing everything she had told me, I realized that part of what I had felt then was shame. I felt foolish for needing to be reminded about reintroducing something so fundamental into my daily considerations. In my quest to clarify how to approach spirituality as a future provider, I recognized that I had been ignoring its place in my own life.

My struggle is one shared by the medical field at large.

Throughout much of history, medicine rested almost solely within the domain of spirituality.[1] People went to their pastors and healers for prayers and rituals to free them of their afflictions. Before there were germs, there were demons that needed casting out. It was understood that care of the body and care of the spirit were inexorably linked. Until the rise of science slowly began to transplant medicine from the world of souls into the world of biochemistry and physiology, healing and spirituality were melded together as one.

There is no doubt that there have been many benefits from this paradigm shift. With scientific advancements came cures and treatments that the healers of antiquity could have never imagined. However, these advances may have also come at the cost of appreciating a holistic approach to health. How pitiful is it when a profession which was once completely focused on healing the whole person must now devote entire conferences and countless seminars to finding ways of injecting it back into both its practitioners and the people they serve?

In modern times, this disconnect is often bridged by the chaplaincy and pastoral care team. I understood this when I first reached out to Reverend Johnson. I hoped that she would be able to shed light on her profession and provide insights on the role of spirituality in medicine.

Going into the call, I could recognize when a consult to a chaplain might be warranted, but I didn't exactly know what the job entailed. I was surprised when one of the first things Reverend Johnson spoke about was how her religious training and background in the Christian spiritual tradition informed her practice but did not take away from who she was able to help. She discussed encounters with people from all backgrounds while within the hospital, ranging from devout Christians all the way to lifelong atheists. She pointed out that every person has a spiritual core that responds to the idea that they have a place in this world, even if that core is not recognized by one of the major religious traditions.

One story that stood out to me was her encounter with a very ill patient who had been referred to pastoral services but did not hold a specific religious creed. The patient's source of spiritual connectedness lay in her appreciation of nature and the beauty of the world around her. Instead of walking through scripture or wrestling with the afterlife, Reverend Johnson recalled sitting with the patient and spending time bringing some peace to her by meditating on the strength and stillness of trees and the Earth. In my opinion, this encounter embodies the role of the chaplain for many patients: chaplains support the part of patients that cannot be reached with medicines, surgeries or analytics.

As Reverend Johnson put it, one of the most important roles of the chaplain is to simply be present with patients. This principle provides the undercurrent on top of which each chaplain's specific theological concentration can build. When these skills are used in tandem, it allows chaplains to serve as symbols that signal to patients they have permission to be human in the moment. A chaplain can become the hand that beckons patients to feel their fears, doubts and frustrations as well as their joys and gratitude. Chaplains offer the presence of someone who will not only refrain from judgement but who will also be by their side as they feel.

Chaplains are also responsible for their more familiar role of tending to people at the end of their lives. Reverend Johnson spoke of a number of heartbreaking experiences she had with patients over the years. She recounted the countless hours she spent sitting with patients and their families, trying to support them as a loved one transitioned out of life. I was struck by how people like her could endure the weight of so many lives day after day and not find themselves buried underneath waves of despair or slowly falling victim to existential crises.

When I asked how she copes with the emotion and the weight of her work, she pointed to her personal spirituality. She explained that inherent in her beliefs is both a calling to service and the reassurance that there is a higher power in charge of everything that is going on. Recognizing that not all providers are religious, she explained that inside most health care providers is a set of beliefs and values that motivate them to wake up in the morning and do their best work for their patients. In her opinion, one of the keys to avoiding burnout and handling those difficult days is to lean on these beliefs. Striving towards deep-seated values brings a kind of fulfillment that is life-giving and not predicated on grades, money, status, or any of the other common distractors in life.

She also pointed out the importance of having people in her life that could support her. It would almost guarantee burnout to hear and see the things that she did on a daily basis and not have anyone with whom she could debrief or decompress. For her, fellow chaplains and a few specially chosen friends served as her support. For the heaviest issues, she advocated seeking formal therapy, a helpful tool that is slowly losing stigma in society but remains a largely untapped resource, especially among provider-types who feel that they have to be "strong" (whatever that means) in order to be successful.

As I continued to probe for advice, she made a special effort to explain that her process of handling the emotionally taxing aspects of medicine is an approach that would benefit all health care providers, including medical students and physicians. We both agreed that the nature of caregiving combined with the heavy work demands of medicine (or medical school) creates an environment where it can become easy to forget about ourselves and our own needs. To combat this, she recommended the daily (as needed or "PRN") timeout where a person takes anywhere from a few seconds to a few minutes to stop, breathe and become more present in the moment. This can take the form of formal meditation, or it can be as simple as taking a moment of silence to check in with yourself and feel whatever emotions or thoughts are alive inside of you at the time.

"Before you are a medical student or doctor or nurse, you're a person," she told me about two-thirds of the way through our call. It was a sentiment that I had heard many other times, but it carried much more weight when hearing it from someone who was so invested in the truth at the core of that statement. We often forget that when something traumatic occurs while on duty (such as witnessing a death), it impacts us beyond our roles as health care providers or students and forms an impression on the person underneath the titles. We invest time into patching the hurt inflicted on our professional selves but stop short of healing the whole person once we have reached a certain level of functionality. As Reverend Johnson underscored throughout our conversation, this approach is woefully incomplete.

To turn to metaphor, we all tend to our lives like gardeners to fruit-bearing trees. If we only ever care for it enough to be fruitful but never take time to examine the roots and the soil, our trees are doomed to never be as tall, as productive, or as long lasting as they can be.

At the end of the call, I thanked her for her prayers and insight. As I laid my phone down and began to quietly reflect on her words, I was saddened by how seldom conversations like ours took place. Part of me cannot help but see some of the blame for this lying at the feet of our institutions. Everyone jokes and pokes one another with sarcastic elbows when we are forced to sit in a mandatory wellness lecture, and we lack buy-in because we can feel its tacked-on nature, even by the most well-meaning institutions.

In a field dominated by the sterility of modern science and idolatry of the bottom-line, it is no surprise that being concerned for the immaterial part of all of us becomes an obligation rather than a truly integrated component of our education and workplace. As I mentioned previously, there are efforts to change this, but I doubt we will ever fully escape the after effects of that first divorce between science and spirituality.

Society at large also holds some of this blame. It makes the twofold mistake of equating spirituality with religion and equating religion with mysticism and superstition. Lost in this logic is the truth that to understand spirituality is to understand what motivates, worries and comforts people at their deepest levels. For this reason, I believe that it is key for health care providers (and their superiors) to realize that appreciating the whole person, including their spiritual side, is the only way to care for people from a truly grounded position.

The transcendence represented in the concept of the soul is the same transcendence that allows a health care worker to care for all kinds of different people. I implore my fellow medical students and future colleagues to not forget this as they strive to become better practitioners in the world. I hope they join me in this difficult but fulfilling journey to attempt to practice soulful medicine.

—

Author's note: I wrote much of this before the COVID pandemic descended upon the world and brought life to a halt. In the midst of so much uncertainty and panic, I think it is even more paramount to take time to explore or express whatever form of spirituality that people believe. The only way to weather a storm is to have a shelter strong enough to stay stable in the winds. Regardless of whether that is a traditional religious practice or your own self-discovered beliefs, now is the time to remember and lean on those beliefs — for our own sake in the middle of this and for our health once this has passed.

Reimagining #MedEd

•

progress

Life as Chimera: When Life Combines With Itself

January 23, 2020

George E. Tsourdinis
University of Illinois College of Medicine, Peoria
Class of 2021

LAMASSU, SPHINX, GANESHA, qilin, centaurs, griffins: amalgams of human-animal species have been mythologized, depicted and deified throughout the history of human civilization. These hybrid species, known collectively as chimeras from the eponymous ancient Greek myth of a lion-goat hybrid, arose from the wellspring of human imagination and creativity. With modern advancements in biotechnology, however, chimeras of a sort are less a myth and more of a reality.

Genetically engineered human pluripotent stem cells (hPSCs) implanted into an evolutionarily-related, nonhuman animal embryo can be considered modern day, corporal chimeras. The concept of chimeras has transcended myth and is now emerging as a tangible, biological spectacle that has been touted to solve the organ transplant shortage and bridge the gap between in vivo animal testing and human clinical research models.

Such powerful research does not come without objections, though. Many arguments against developing chimeras span the gamut of moral ideologies and engage medical ethics. In order for future physicians to grapple with thorny bioethical dilemmas surrounding concepts like chimera research, we need not only understand their biochemical and clinical mechanisms, but we must also delve into the philosophy and art surrounding these issues. Analyzing the histories of chimera art and mythology alongside moral philosophies can aid in comprehending the full context of said debate before forging our own opinions.

Chimeras, like hPSCs, have much potential in enhancing human health, and they are already becoming a possibility in the early stages of research (the first human-pig chimeras were created successfully early in 2017).[1] One group has even successfully grown healthy mouse-derived pancreases in rats, which were then harvested and transplanted into diabetic mice. They successfully secreted insulin and thereby reversed the diabetes of the mice.[2]

Given such sparks of success, chimera technology has seen a dramatic rise in popularity — and dissent. In 2015, the National Institutes of Health (NIH) issued a funding moratorium on chimera research until the bioethics were better resolved. In August of 2016, the NIH lifted this same moratorium from chimera research under the stipulation that an ethics oversight committee would monitor the research.[3] However, legislation is continually being drafted to prevent such research, and the opposition present in the literature is even more deafening.

What forms the basis of this formerly-banned and now-restricted research? We can look along diverse philosophical veins to see where the discomfort in chimera research originates. One such vein is the "Unnaturalness Argument," which was supported by a prominent 20th-century philosopher of biology, Hans Jonas. Deeming chimeras as "unnatural" and thus wrong, Jonas claims an inherent disgust evoked by moral intuition that "produce[s] an involuntary shudder" — colloquially dubbed the 'yuck factor.' The underlying thesis of the Unnaturalness Argument is that chimeras transgress some natural divide between humans and nonhumans, and that issues them with a moral prohibition. To Jonas, the very "interchange of genetic material between animals and man" would summon "ancient, forgotten terms such as 'sacrilege' and 'abomination.'"[4]

Still, the aversive reflexes evoked from the concept of the "admixture" of an animal and human could be considered an over-inflated concern by some. In discussing gene therapy technologies, contemporary philosopher and biophysicist, Henri Atlan, paints the Unnaturalness Argument as "irrational fears which derive from misunderstandings in biology, and are compounded by the effects of popular creations of fiction, such as Frankenstein's monster." In that same report, Atlan recognizes that, perhaps that it is not simply unjustified fear or "merely a fear of the unknown that engenders caution, but also a recognition that the ability to modify the genetic endowment of human beings ... in touching the gene, therefore is touching the essence of life."

Here, Atlan conceives of the implicit "playing god" phobia — or "master of the hereditary model," as Jonas refers to it.[5] Importantly, Atlan points out that the "essence of life" is a "wooly" or vague notion, one that biomedical ethics must eschew from and adopt a more "pragmatic" analysis of each instance of bioethical debate by "[analyzing] the specific potentially dangerous or undesirable effects."

One example of such a "pragmatic" analysis lies in the most-feared scenario of chimeric organisms: the situation in which hPSCs tread off the genetic lineage intended by researchers and into a neural fate, where hPSCs either form a mosaic of human-animal neural tissue or completely pervade the nervous system of the host organism. Today, despite significant progress in (epi)genetic knowledge, the issue with chimeras is that scientists have still not elucidated how hPSCs precisely migrate in utero. Therefore, it has been postulated that hPSCs implanted into animals could diverge from their original coaxing to instead take hold in the areas that are destined to become embryonic neural tissue. Assuming this (e.g. human-pig) chimera was brought to full term, what would hypothetically result is a newborn pig with a genetically-human central nervous system.

Questions pour forth: does the chimeric animal achieve a sort of moral status? Does the chimera have the same rights that a human would? Can the animal cognize as a human would, and would experimentation/organ harvesting on the animal thus be considered unethical due to the sensations and suffering it would undergo? The existence of borderline human-nonhuman chimeras could generate moral and ontological confusion. But consider how the modern surgical procedure of xenotransplanting a porcine heart valve is morally acceptable for many patients (save for patients of religious backgrounds that prohibit the consumption of porcine food products, namely Islam and Judaism).[6] Perhaps it is the possession of a specifically human central nervous system, which provides sensation and cognition, by a nonhuman animal that truly enlivens the 'grotesque' reaction to chimeras in some.

When discussing chimeras in scientific research, it is rare that we consider our very selves to be chimeras, too, just shaped by the different mechanism of natural selection. According to endosymbiotic theory, our own mitochondria derive from an oxidative prokaryote that was engulfed by a larger prokaryotic host cell, essentially forming a symbiotic chimera of sorts that ultimately evolved to power complex, multicellular organisms like Homo sapiens.[7] As 'natural' chimeras ourselves, selected over time to think and create and debate, we are responsible for directing the course of synthetic chimera research and its potential use in the future of biomedicine.

Blaise Pascal once proclaimed in his Pensées, "What a chimera then is man! What a novelty! What a monster, what a chaos, what a contradiction, what a prodigy!" [8] Just as Pascal invokes the clashing qualities of humankind's essence as chimeric, so too are scientists and bioethicists as divided on chimera research today. Certainly, the incomprehensibility about what constitutes life and what factors make humans human is grounds for some to hold an instinctive aversion to promoting chimera research. But the utilitarian benefits that could spring from chimera biomedical research must not be ignored either. As biotechnology progresses rapidly, future physicians will have to trod the murky path of new bioethical dilemmas with both the medical humanities and scientific medicine as our guiding lights.

REIMAGINING #MEDED

Well, It Happened: Step 1 Will Become Pass/Fail
February 21, 2020

Pranav Reddy, MD, MPA at Yale New Haven Hospital
Kunal K. Sindhu, MD at Mount Sinai Medical Center
Bryan Carmody, MD, MPH at Children's Hospital of the King's Daughters

LAST WEEK, THE United States Medical Licensing Examination (USMLE) announced that Step 1, the first of three required licensing examinations for medical trainees, will stop reporting three-digit scores and instead report only a pass/fail designation as early as January 2022.[1] The three-digit scoring systems for Step 2 Clinical Knowledge (CK) and Step 3, and the pass/fail system for Step 2 Clinical Skills, will remain unchanged.

In explaining its decision to change the Step 1 scoring system, the USMLE noted that its co-sponsors, the National Board of Medical Examiners (NBME) and the Federation of State Medical Boards (FSMB), "believe that changing Step 1 score reporting to pass/fail can help reduce some of the current overemphasis on USMLE performance, while also retaining the ability of medical licensing authorities to use the exam for its primary purpose of medical licensure eligibility."[1] We have also made similar arguments advocating for a shift to a pass/fail scoring system in the past due to concerns regarding the three-digit score's pernicious effect on medical curricula, medical student well-being and its misuse in selecting candidates for specialty training.[2-6]

It is only fair that we give the USMLE and its corporate sponsors credit for making the right decision. As we noted in a piece for *in-House* prior to the Invitational Conference on USMLE Scoring last year, there were plenty of reasons, including glaring financial conflicts of interest and worrisome written comments from the leaders of the NBME and FSMB, to suspect that the USMLE and its sponsors would maintain the status quo.[3,7,8] Ultimately, the harms of maintaining the "Step 1 Climate" became too great to ignore, even for the test's corporate sponsors.[9]

Since the news broke, many have reacted with strong feelings.[10] Many medical students, residents, and faculty are overjoyed, viewing the change as a long overdue course correction for medical education. Others have strongly criticized the decision, arguing that it will remove an essential "objective" metric for selecting medical students for residencies and harm individuals from international medical schools and less prominent American medical schools.[11-14]

These criticisms are not entirely without merit but ignore the realities of how we got here. USMLE Step 1, a multiple choice question test of basic science knowledge, was never intended to be used as it is today. The reliance on Step 1 scores in resident selection was a decision rooted in convenience, not evidence; since all students have Step 1 scores available by the time they apply for residency, Step 1 scores can be used as a "filter" to reduce a mountain of applications to a manageable pile. However, the skills required to score well on Step 1 are not the same as those required to become a good doctor.[15]

Step 1 scores are objective, but that doesn't mean they are meaningful, precise, or predictive of residency success. All program directors would agree that a Step 1 score of 250 is higher than a score of 235. But does that mean that an applicant with the former score will become a better resident than the latter? In fact, because the standard error of difference for USMLE Step 1 is 8 points, scores must differ by 16 points or more for a program director to conclude with 95% confidence that there is even a significant difference in test performance between the two applicants.[16]

On the other hand, who will be a better resident: a student with an extensive research background, or one who started a free clinic? A student who is the first in their family to attend college, or a member of the Gold Humanism Honor Society? Deciding which of these applicants is more likely to succeed in a particular residency program requires a human judgment, and different programs will likely make different decisions. Outsourcing that decision to a three-digit score was convenient but prevents program directors from viewing applicants as individuals and making mission-based selection decisions.

Lastly, while a few international medical graduates (IMGs) with high Step 1 scores and ambitions to practice medicine in the United States have benefited from the scored Step 1 system, the truth is that the vast majority have not.[13] Average Step 1 scores and match rates for IMGs lag significantly behind those for American allopathic and osteopathic students.[17] The majority of United States residency programs do not consider non-U.S. citizen IMGs, and IMGs are especially rare in the most selective specialties.[18,19] As it currently stands, as Dr. Benjamin Mazer has pointed out, the school from which a medical student graduates significantly impacts where he or she matches. Making Step 1 pass/fail does not change that unpleasant truth.

To some degree, however, these criticisms highlight a larger point: Step 1's transformation to pass/fail should not be viewed as the end in itself. There is a larger root rot in the way in which candidates are selected for medical residencies. Today, many physicians do not practice in the field that most appealed to them, privilege and race often impede many from training in medicine, and medical education often focuses on esoteric basic science facts in an effort to teach to the test rather than emphasize the larger art and science of medicine.[20-27] As a result, programs screen and select candidates based on narrow and arbitrary measures unrelated to their ability to practice as a doctor, and a small group of applicants take up an outsized number of interview slots.[28] If the ultimate outcome of this transition is to emphasize yet another imperfect, albeit more clinically relevant, numeric metric like Step 2 CK, another arms race will ensue, and an opportunity for transformative change would be missed.

What would transformative change look like? We believe residency programs should move away from the idea that any one-size-fits-all numeric metric can identify the applicants best suited for success in every specialty and program and instead should embrace holistic review.[29] Students from international and less-prestigious medical schools rightly point out that they may not have the same access to C.V. — boosting research opportunities or high-profile letters of recommendation as their peers at more prestigious schools. But it is only by considering applicants as individuals that "distance traveled" and success with the available resources can even be considered. No objective measure can do that for us.

Considering an applicant's experiences, personal attributes, and academic qualifications in combination will likely better match applicants with the right residency program. But unless we couple the pass/fail Step 1 with efforts to limit the volume of applications programs receive, program directors will gravitate to another numeric screening metric out of necessity. Accordingly, applicant and interview caps, lotteries, and early acceptance programs to residency should all be considered as ways to stop application fever and make applying to residency more fair and rational.[30,31] These proposed changes are just the start, and the next two years provide ample opportunity to rethink how we teach medical students and select them for residency.

Ending Step 1 mania was a great step forward for medical education in America. But the time for change is just beginning.

Unpacking the "Insult" of Being Called a Nurse as a Female Physician

March 2, 2020

Jessa Fogel
Vanderbilt University School of Medicine
Class of 2022

IT'S A COMMON SCENARIO: a male medical student and a female resident walk into a patient's room together, and the patient automatically assumes that the man is the doctor and the woman is the nurse. Despite the fact that more women than men enrolled in U.S. medical schools in 2019, female medical students, residents and even attending physicians are far more likely to be mistaken for nurses than their male counterparts — women of color even more so.[1] As a female medical student myself, I like to joke that if I had a dollar for every time someone in the hospital called me a nurse, I could pay off all my student loans.

This is a problem. Certainly, with the myriad of roles and responsibilities in a hospital setting, having your position constantly mistaken for another is not only frustrating, but it can also compromise patient care due to miscommunication between team members. However, I worry a bit when I hear conversations among female physicians going something like this: "...and then, he called me a nurse! Can you imagine? Um, excuse me, I did not go through four years of medical school to be called a *nurse*."

Can we stop for a moment and consider why being called a nurse is insulting to female physicians and medical students?

It's not just because it is factually incorrect; rather, it is an incorrect assumption based on a stereotype. A two-second glance at my badge could confirm my role in the hospital, but many people don't even take that time, which alone is sufficient grounds for my irritation. Furthermore, the convenience of the stereotype is born from the assumption that a woman in scrubs couldn't possibly have gone through the extensive training required to become a doctor. This, of course, is offensive and must be addressed.

But what really bothers me about this scenario, in addition to the often incorrect assumptions made about a woman's title in the hospital, is the implicit notion that female physicians are working harder than their nursing counterparts to challenge gender stereotypes. There is a belief that the "successful" women in medicine, the ones who are shattering glass ceilings and closing gender gaps in the workplace, are the physicians — not the nurses. For example, as Dr. Megan Lemay writes in an article originally published on KevinMD.com, "To me, it feels like we've just splintered the shell of this previously male-dominated field. Being called 'nurse' reminds me of the enormous gender gap I have yet to cross. Overpowering gender stereotypes will take more than outnumbering the men in our field." [2] I doubt many people in medicine today need convincing that female doctors face a preposterous amount of sexism throughout their training (but here's an article on the subject anyway).[3]

But we must realize that the field of nursing also faces challenges with regards to gender discrimination — albeit in different ways than those seen in medicine. Unlike doctoring, nursing has always been dominated by women.[4] And these women in nursing have had their work cut out for them in order to elevate their profession into what it is today. Nursing has risen from an unskilled position requiring no formal education prior to the 19th century to a hugely diverse field with opportunities for advanced practice degrees, research, and teaching.[5]

Unfortunately, despite all of these advances, nurses are still struggling against gender bias in the workplace. The very fact that male nurses face judgement and stigma over their pursuit of a "feminine career" says quite a lot about the perceptions of female-dominated professions.[6] As a result of traditional views of women as subordinates, particularly in the health care setting, nurses often face disrespect and discrimination from physicians.[7]

And still, despite the predominance of women in nursing, there remains gender bias within the field, not just outside of it. Just as female physicians lament the deficit of women in leadership positions in medicine, surveys have shown that in the United Kingdom, male nurses are roughly twice as likely to hold certain leadership positions in the hospital.[8] Somehow, female nurses are even fighting a gender pay gap, according to the 2018 Nursing Salary Research Report.[9] Suffice to say that although they may not be breaking into a male-dominated field, nurses — as professional women — are nevertheless fighting gender stereotypes just as their female physician counterparts are in the hopes that their voices will be heard and respected as fellow care providers.[10]

As female doctors and doctors-to-be, when we're mistaken for nurses, it's frustrating to feel like our work to enter the field of medicine has gone unrecognized. But this frustration ought not to mask the fact that nurses, too, are fighting battles of their own when it comes to gender discrimination. Women in medicine and nursing, let's all shatter glass ceilings together without tearing each other down. Let's stop making assumptions, and start treating each other with the respect we all deserve as members of a health care team.

IN-TRAINING: 2020 IN OUR WORDS

More Than Skin Deep: Underrepresentation of Brown and Black Skin in Medical Education

August 1, 2020

Maiya Smith and Tyler Thorne
John A. Burns School of Medicine in Honolulu, Hawaii
Class of 2022

MEDICINE IS A DISCIPLINE that claims to be based on empirical and scientific truth about human nature. Instead, its knowledge and practice are often steeped in biases like racism. For example, medicine was used in the nineteenth century to justify slavery due to the "biologically inherent superiority" of White races.[1] Dr. Thomas Hamilton was a Southern physician in the nineteenth century who used torturous medical experiments on slaves in an attempt to prove false narratives on physiological differences between the skin of Black and White people.[2] One of his experiments included blistering the skin of slaves to "prove" their skin was thicker. And the Tuskegee syphilis trials leave a long legacy of medical mistrust.

Many racial biases still exist and affect the care of people of color, especially Black patients. A 2016 survey found that about one-third of medical students and residents surveyed believed that Black people have thicker skin than their non-Hispanic White counterparts (NHWC).[3] This pervasive and racist idea contributes to the inadequate pain management of Black patients and is sadly not the only myth that is still perpetuated in the realm of dermatology.

Dermatological health disparities have long been well-documented in people of color: non-white patients have higher rates of morbidity and mortality associated with dermatologic disease as compared to their NHWC.[4] Additionally, under-recognition of erythema migrans in Lyme disease has resulted in increased rates of late manifestations in Black patients.[5] Black children, based on race alone, are also less likely to see a medical provider for their eczema in the ambulatory setting.[5] These disparities may have to do with the fact that representation of race and skin tone in medical textbooks are predominantly skewed towards White skin tones.[6] As a result, inclusivity in dermatological education is long overdue. Given that dermatology is the second least diverse specialty in medicine, action should also be taken to reduce this educational disparity.[7] Medical students themselves have already begun to advocate for this change.

The White Coats for Black Lives organization was created in 2014 in response to the non-indictment of officers responsible for the deaths of Michael Brown and Eric Garner. Medical students across the country have more recently flocked to social media, posting images of themselves with the hashtag #whitecoats4blacklives after the police murder of George Floyd. At the time of writing this piece, a petition advocating for medical schools to include Black and other minority representation in clinical teaching had amassed 189,120 signatures.[8] Students are even taking to journal submissions, writing about their personal experiences with discriminatory medical education and recommending avenues for change.[9] In an effort to decolonize medical education, one passionate Black medical student wrote a book called *Mind The Gap*, a handbook of clinical signs on Black and Brown skin.[10] Through action, students have shown that they will no longer take part in discriminatory medical education that not only promotes systemic racism but also hinders their ability to be competent physicians.

One further solution is to increase exposure to pathology on Brown and Black skin amongst medical students, as this is proven to increase confidence in diagnosing a variety of dermatological diseases.[11] In addition to diversifying images of dermatological pathologies in textbooks, the field can also diversify research to identify potential racial or ethnic disparities in the diagnosis and treatment of dermatologic diseases. These changes are especially needed given that the projected growth rate of minority populations is increasing every year. The non-Caucasian U.S. population could be approximately 48% by the year 2050.[12] Many of us become physicians to help our communities; yet, only learning from textbooks often steeped in the racist legacy of medicine is insufficient. And so, medical education must change the curriculum to ensure proper representation of darker skin tones.

Other specialties have already distinguished themselves as leaders in health inequities. In fact, family medicine (FM) was born during the time of the Civil Rights movement and Vietnam War protests as part of the "countercultural" movement with social responsibility at its core.[13] At the root of FM is the understanding that economic, social and cultural forces impact access to health care and that it is paramount to acknowledge these forces to provide health care for all people. As such, FM strives to continuously address the social determinants of health and reaffirm its unique position in influencing needed changes in health care. It is important for the field of dermatology to similarly emulate FM's goal to alleviate health disparities because, as it currently stands, dermatology only caters to a small population of primarily light-skinned individuals. With a more comprehensive education that includes Black and Brown skin, dermatology can further embrace the Hippocratic Oath and appropriately treat all patients knowing that skin diseases may present differently on various skin tones.

Given the current political change in our nation and the more ubiquitous momentum behind the Black Lives Matter movement, dermatologic medical education should take this opportunity to reflect on its own implicit bias and include Black and Brown skin images in the teaching of dermatological conditions. Actively including more representation in dermatological textbooks is crucial to dismantling internalized racist beliefs that students already consciously or unconsciously hold, and to increasing their awareness of how diseases can present on different skin tones. This is more than just a matter of diversity; it is a matter of providing equitable life-saving care.

REIMAGINING #MEDED

You're Not a Bold, Knowledgeable Medical Student — You're Just White
July 25, 2020

Nat Mulkey
Boston University School of Medicine
Class of 2021

IT WAS A THURSDAY NIGHT, and I was with my two friends, Jess and Kevin, on the dark road back to Boston. We were on our surgery rotation in a distant town. During the week, we cohabited in a bare-necessities house near the hospital. As the only one with a car, it became my routine to wait until everyone's long shifts were over and drive everyone back. We tended to fill these rides with conversation, the topic of which was often our experiences on the wards. Tonight was not any different. Trying to keep my tired eyes on the road, I just listened to Jess and Kevin talk.

The conversation turned to the concept of "imposter syndrome" — that feeling of not belonging in a space you were accepted into institutionally. Kevin described how all of third year has been draining in an unexpected way. He went on to say it has been hard for him to be himself completely, or to feel like he fits in. Jess validated this and brought up that it probably had a lot to do with how they were raised.

For context, Kevin is Vietnamese and Jess is Chinese. They got to discussing the similarities in how they were brought up — how respect for parents and other older family members was paramount and manifested in actions, not just words. For them, as children, it was not socially acceptable to speak up to or question a senior family member. The connection between this upbringing and their ability to navigate the archaic hierarchy of medicine was not lost on them. It was not easy for them to speak up or chime in during rounds, to offer their knowledge or perspective to a group of seniors.

At that point, a lightbulb went off in my own inner monologue: of course.

Before witnessing this conversation, if you had asked me how it feels to be a part of the medical team, I would have said, "easy." I would have bragged about my ability to speak up to superiors — how I easily fight for a plan others initially disagree with or bring up more radical advocacy notions that question someone's management. These are things I have come to hold as core aspects of my personality. In listening to Jess and Kevin, I realized how ignorant that really was.

What I have been interpreting as character traits are products of my White cultural upbringing. In my life, less emphasized were the values brought up by Kevin and Jess in the car that night — that of respect for authority and the importance of group cohesion over the needs of the individual. While I am not implying this is the situation for all students of Asian descent, it was a clear cultural difference between me and these two friends. My upbringing placed more value on individual expression, achievement, and choice. From childhood, I have been primed to speak up and demonstrate my ability, regardless of who I am speaking to. In fact, it has been encouraged. And this has served me well on the wards.

Feeling that my voice is wanted and even necessary in the clinical setting does more than ease my experience, it offers tangible benefits. To understand how, it is necessary to understand how we are assessed.

Medical students receive "clinical grades" that transform their performance in the clinical setting into a numerical or categorical term. Some components of these evaluations include knowledge, measured by our ability to diagnose and plan for a patient's care. In practice, the moments to showcase our skills are not clearly defined. So, demonstration of knowledge involves both successful identification of those moments and what many physicians label as "confidence" to seize the moment. Over and over again I have heard seniors tell students, "It doesn't really matter what you say for a diagnosis or plan, just say it with confidence." This confidence emphasized by evaluators, who are responsible for our grades, is not an objective measure of ability, but instead the result of how comfortable a medical student is in a space. And if you are White, I promise you are probably a lot more comfortable than a student who is not.

You are more comfortable because you are familiar with the culture of medicine, and how to navigate it. This is because, in many ways, the culture of medicine is White culture. White physicians make up 56% of the workforce, more than any other race or ethnicity.[1] I have been on a variety of medical teams during my third year, but it is safe to say the majority of those teams were White people. I knew I moved through these spaces easily for many reasons, but being White is a big one that needs to be said out loud. And when you look and feel more comfortable in a space, it is easier to perform "well," or to sound confident. This is directly related to what academic medicine characterizes as "objective" evaluations of students, and there is data to support this.

A study summarizing 6,000 Medical Student Performance Evaluations found that White students were more likely to be described as "standout" and their abilities to be "exceptional" and "outstanding."[2] Black students, meanwhile, were more likely to be described as "competent." They found that medical students who were not White received lower grades than

White students in most of their clinical clerkships. These clinical grades carry weight — not only do potential residencies see them, they are also used to select for prestigious society memberships such as Alpha Omega Alpha. White students are six times more likely to be induced into Alpha Omega Alpha compared to Black students and two times more likely compared to Asian students.[3]

As we neared our exit, I shared my own experience with Jess and Kevin, detailing my surprise at never having developed the dreaded "imposter syndrome." I told them how listening to their conversation made me realize, and more critically evaluate, the reason behind this. I know a lot about White privilege and the socioeconomic implications of it. Medical schools actually elucidate the results of White privilege by teaching us about racial disparities. But we rarely discuss the huge ways in which the predominant White culture of medicine diminishes the subjective experiences of minority students and their "objective" evaluations.

This moment in the car on the way home was an important reminder of that.

But this reminder needs to go further. There are many ways in which I, as a White medical student, can improve this problem. For example, I can make note of when I need to pipe down and instead help amplify another student's voice while in the clinical setting. I can support students who have adverse experiences due to their race by joining their voice when they speak to the administration. The reflection I engaged in in the car was a passive happenstance, but active and continued reflection, instead of when prompted by students of color, is critically important. Additionally, it is crucial we support institutional-level change. For instance some schools are suspending their affiliation with the Alpha Omega Alpha.[4] Supporting movements to end metrics that favor the White medical students, like the USMLE STEP scoring system, is another way.[5] This is by no means an exhaustive list, but these are tangible steps that remove barriers for students of color. There is a lot of work to be done to make medical education — particularly in the clinical realm — a safer space for our non-White students.

This car ride was a reminder that the first step is always the same: sit back and listen.

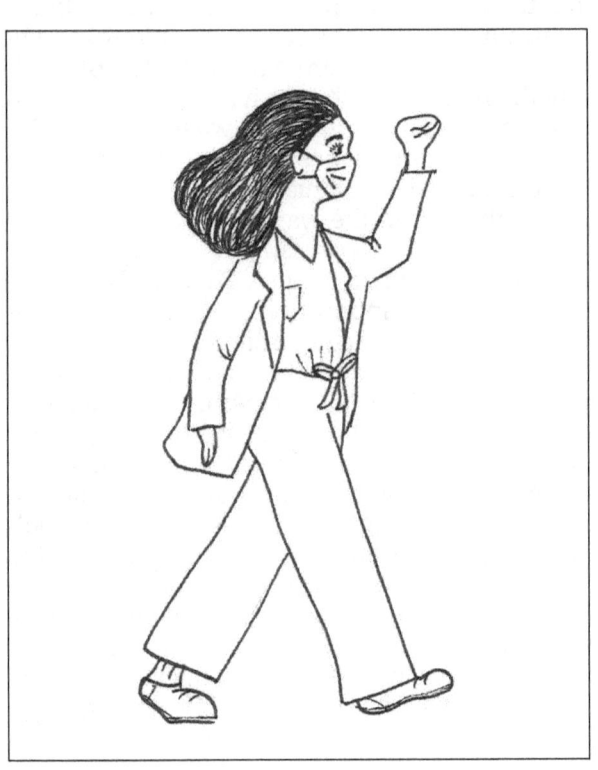

Advocacy: This Is Our Lane

•

racism

The Autopsy Report of Mr. George Floyd

June 16, 2020

Amal Cheema
Geisel School of Medicine at Dartmouth
Class of 2023

The Autopsy Report[I] of Mr. George Floyd:[II] Mechanical Asphyxia[III,IV]

—

[I] *There was more than one objective report on homicide.* The first headline — cardiopulmonary arrest, positive for COVID-19. Followed by public outrage: we saw without prodding or proximity, we knew without license or degree, we heard and we witnessed all that his body testified: the crush of the knee looting air from lungs, the drowning of his pulmonary parenchyma, his cries of "I can't breathe." The second — mechanical asphyxia. There is no justice in muddy medical terminology or listservs of forensic coroners who disagree. The third report has yet to be typeset but it will name — racism, as the cause of death.

[II] He was a tall man with tall dreams, out buying at the local grocery. *For more information, please see this non-comprehensive list:* Tony, Breonna, Ahmaud, Trayvon, Michael, Kionte … and Dante, Ezell, Michael, John, Eric, Emmett. *For a medical directory, please read:* of the unethical practice of an antebellum "father of modern gynecology," of the procurement of Ms. Lacks' cells, of the execution of the Study on Syphilis. Ibid., slavery.

[III] A Black man of his age, his chances of dying were already high. Experts were surprised to see he had survived COVID, as we know that takes more Black lives. If not virus or brutality, consider a health disparity: too much blood sugar, too much blood pressure, too much of another nationally notifiable, historically accepted disease. Assuredly, upon further questioning, we may comfortably suggest lifestyle, socioeconomic status, environment, or other factors as immutable, statistical context. What shall go unaddressed is covert, overt systemic oppression in which we remain comfortably complicit.

[IV] Pressed for time, the report shall be quick to conclude: For eight minutes and forty-six seconds, Mr. Floyd could not breathe with a knee on his neck, and thus met his untimely, unconscionable death.

Images of Violence Unravel Us — And Our Communities

June 5, 2020

Anna Ayala
Oregon Health and Science University
Class of 2023

THREE MONTHS AGO, two white men slayed Ahmaud Arbery. One of the men who committed this murder shared the gruesome video with local media, under the assumption that it would absolve him of the crime.[1] One month after Mr. Arbery's murder, the video went viral, being shared thousands of times as a plea to the criminal legal system: find these men and bring them to justice.

Ten nights ago, a white Minneapolis police officer murdered George Floyd while two other officers restrained him and another watched.[2] Like the video of Mr. Arbery's murder, this video went viral, giving millions of people unfettered access to the last minutes of Mr. Floyd's precious life.

Importantly, *this viewership does not come without offense.*

Images of deeply graphic violence grant non-Black individuals a permit into the reality of police brutality against Black individuals. These 'permits' traumatize the Black community while simultaneously allowing the non-Black holder the right to participate as a transitory viewer. Non-Black individuals can neither begin to understand the Black experience in America nor understand the relationship between the Black body and state-sanctioned police. We can only passively view the video of Mr. Arbery's murder: pause, rewind, replay it. We can inquire, ruminate, and speak at length but only from a place of privilege. We may watch with fury, if only for an instant.

Non-Black people can turn away. We can shift our gaze towards the unforgivable violence against Mr. Floyd or flee from it when we are uncomfortable. These images only benefit those of us who do not experience systemic police brutality — those who are shielded from the violent arm of racism that devalues and erases Black individuals and communities. Our haphazard use of these photographs and videos are rooted in a long history of public ownership of the Black body, and thereby preserve the American tradition of criminalization and desensitization.

But this is not the case for the Black community. Mr. Floyd's murder is not momentary. It is cemented in video; his pain and suffering calcified into the skeleton of our nation's dark history, haunting Black lives daily.

It is a violation of the integrity of another human's life to watch them die in a graphic and violent manner. After all, we rarely observe this phenomenon with non-Black bodies in our media. And in medicine, we make many attempts to preserve the dignity of our patients in death and dying. The recent public murders call into question the responsibility of our gaze. Why is it that the only way to mobilize non-Black individuals to observe, recognize, and act against racism is to watch a Black man die? We must do better.

For six nights, protests in downtown Portland culminated in front of the Multnomah County Justice Center, a holding cell for temporary jailing and a testament to the inextricable history of injustice inflicted upon Black America. The protests and destruction highlight the rage, despair, and hurt that flows within and throughout the Black community in Portland. In a city with such an undeniable history of racism and subsequent erasure, these events were a consequence of systemic violence and the anguish that follows.[3]

We should not need to view videos of Black individuals suffering or in pain in order to mobilize. Others, unrecorded and alone, die by the hands of our state at an unimaginable rate. It is time for Americans to turn their gaze away from violent images of Black death and inwards to consider the invisible and blatant ways we uphold white supremacy every single day. We must recognize it in our workplaces, public spaces, and homes — and, importantly, in our clinics and hospitals.

After all, our lives as future physicians are molded by the act of ameliorating suffering. Our patients come to us with bodies shaped by deprivation and trauma. We must understand that this pain is revealed to us in confidence, protected by the venerable patient-physician relationship, and should be treated with grace, respect, and integrity. Just like we consume video-recorded violence, we can be transiently interested in our patient's social circumstances and then look away when we are uncomfortable. We cannot allow this to perpetuate. We must neither passively consume their stories nor ignore them. Instead, we must hold each other accountable. We must recognize that we are bound to our violent history that calls upon us to reckon with a medical establishment that routinely does harm, and to unlearn the cultural logic that devalues Black individuals and their health.

IN-TRAINING: 2020 IN OUR WORDS

This is Water: A Perspective on Race from a White Male

July 26, 2020

Caleb Sokolowski
Wayne State University School of Medicine
Class of 2023

IN HIS GRADUATION SPEECH at Kenyon College in 2005, David Foster Wallace gave a thought-provoking speech that rings true in today's hostile climate.[1] Wallace began with a story: "There are these two young fish swimming along and they happen to meet an older fish swimming the other way, who nods at them and says 'Morning, boys. How's the water?' And the two young fish swim on for a bit, and then eventually one of them looks over at the other and goes 'What the hell is water?'"

As humans, we experience life through a lens that is unique to ourselves. We spend most of our life in a "default setting" and rarely look outside of our natural inclinations to view the world. The way we are raised and our experiences shape this unique lens through which we see reality.

As a White male, there are certain things that I will never understand. I was raised in an upper-middle-class family in a safe neighborhood — one with adequate resources, education and funding. I have never had to live in fear in my community, worry about my safety on my street, or been threatened or condemned because of how I look. My reality is inexplicably shaped by the privilege and opportunities that I have been given. I realize that, to me, racism appears nonexistent because I have not seen it.

But while I have my reality, I, ashamedly, am just beginning to recognize that there are many others who are experiencing life in a dichotomous way. There are some who, because of the color of their skin and the neighborhood they were raised in, have to spend their lives living in fear. Fear of walking on the street. Fear of driving their car. Fear of looking at someone the wrong way.

A few months after receiving my driver's license, I was pulled over by a police officer on my way home from a friend's house for going 14 miles per hour over the speed limit. Not only was I speeding, but it was almost two hours past the Michigan curfew set for new drivers. After spending a few moments talking with the police officer, he told me that for breaking those laws, this incident could go on my public record, and I could have my driver's license revoked for more than a year. To my surprise, however, the officer then told me that while he could enforce the law, he was going to let me go as long as I promised to go straight home and tell my parents what had happened.

I have reflected on this experience many times throughout my life. I had previously rationalized the situation by believing that I had either simply gotten lucky or said the right things during my conversation with the officer. It was not until the national discussions that are developing currently, however, that I began to wonder what would have happened that night if I were in a low-income neighborhood and had a higher concentration of melanin in my skin.

For those of us that do not visibly experience racism, it is so easy to live life in our default setting and ignore the realities that are clear to many around us. This cannot continue. We must find moments to reflect on what we otherwise have a difficult time understanding. Realities like racism that we don't immediately recognize are the hardest to admit and discuss, but they are also pivotal for us to grow as a society that respects and honors all people, regardless of skin color.

While the water I swim in may lead me to think that racism is a thing of the past, I must begin to educate myself on how the inequalities of the past seep into the reality of today. I need to continue to realize that because my family wasn't a victim of mortgage discrimination and pushed to live in certain neighborhoods due to redlining, I have benefited.[2] I need to remind myself that even down to the care my mother received when I was in her womb, I have benefited from the color of my skin.[3]

As future physicians, we take an oath to "do no harm," but if we remain complacent in issues that unquestionably affect the health and wellness of others, then we are not staying true to that promise.[4] While this is a complex problem that will take time and hard work to fix, medical students and physicians must first recognize that there even is a problem and that it needs to be discussed early and often. While we can't change everyone or everything (at least not all at once), we can start by working to shed light on the inequalities seen in the health care system.[5] We can improve our medical education system to include lessons on the systemic racism seen throughout the United States so that it doesn't take a countrywide revolution for us to recognize the water that is all around us.

As I continue to reflect on my privilege and uncover what is not immediately evident to my eyes, I challenge you to do so as well. Zeno, a Greek philosopher, once said, "Man conquers the world by conquering himself." Let us all strive to realize that we are not the center of the universe, that we are merely a drop in the ocean of humanity. A humanity that is not inherently divided by skin color but is united as one human race. Let us think about those whose reality may be starkly different from our own, and let us continue to remind ourselves that "this is water."

IN-TRAINING: 2020 IN OUR WORDS

Physicians' Role in Addressing Racism
November 27, 2020

Swetha Tummala
Boston University School of Medicine
Class of 2024

MERCEDES DROVE TWO HOURS to the nearest health care clinic to get her first physical exam in ten years. I met Mercedes while shadowing primary care physician Dr. L. In the clinic, Mercedes divulged to me how nervous she had been driving in — she knew what the meeting held in store. Her fears were confirmed: just five minutes into her exam, Dr. L advised her, "Mercedes, you have to lose weight."

Mercedes is part of a national epidemic. As of 2016, 40% of Americans are obese.[1] When considering factors that impact an individual's weight, the public and the media tend to focus on individual behavior such as diet and exercise.[2] We may blame individuals like Mercedes, attributing their weight to laziness. "Try harder," Mercedes recounted to me in the clinic, is advice she often hears.

However, this advice is inadequate. Though individual behavior plays a role, it cannot fully explain the striking disparity in the prevalence of obesity by race. Mercedes is a 46-year-old Black woman, and Black/African Americans disproportionately suffer the highest obesity rates — 48% among Black/African Americans compared to 43% among Latinos, 35% among Whites and 12% among Asians.[3] This disparity is especially concerning now since obesity increases the risk of severe illness from COVID-19.[4] The disproportionately high obesity rate among Black/African Americans stems from the broader issue of racism and its impact on the built environment, or the man-made aspects of where one lives.

Mercedes spent months searching for safe, affordable housing in Alabama before settling for her two-bedroom house next to Highway 18. Beginning in the 1930s, the U.S. government refused to grant Black/African Americans housing loans in a policy called redlining, forcing Black/African Americans into poorer neighborhoods.[5] Though redlining has long been banned, its impacts persist. Black/African Americans still form the majority of residents in redlined neighborhoods.[6]

Redlined neighborhoods generally lack access to fresh food, adequate green space and larger hospitals.[7] They face more pollution and violence.[7] With two jobs, a long commute, and two kids, the only downtime Mercedes gets is an hour in the late evenings. However, with few street lights and constant traffic in her neighborhood, she does not feel safe walking outside at night which has greatly limited her physical activity.

As a result of country-wide protests and increased awareness of the disproportionate burden of COVID-19 on racial and ethnic minority groups, more physicians are beginning to recognize the effects of race and racism on health.[8] After Mercedes left the clinic that day, a quiet, low tone replaced Dr. L's usually brassy voice as she talked through the situation with a colleague. Dr. L had felt helpless as she treated Mercedes for high blood pressure and diabetes but knew Mercedes was going back to the same environmental conditions that were causing her ailments.

Some may wonder, is it a physician's duty to address racism? A physician's primary role is to provide the highest quality health care to those in need. However, racial biases can affect the delivery of care, especially in emergency situations.[9] Racism has profound impacts on health, and there are a multitude of ways for physicians to address it in meaningful ways without overburdening themselves. In fact, addressing racism can improve medical care.[9] It can help physicians identify a possible root cause of the health-harming conditions in which a patient may live and can reduce physicians' implicit racial biases, which have been shown to affect quality of care.[10]

Learning how to integrate practices to reduce racial bias and inequity is a process that should start as early as medical school — during hiring, admissions and first-year training. During hiring and admissions, medical schools should aim for racial diversity among students, faculty, staff and administration to help their affiliates meet people from different backgrounds, broaden their perspectives, and practice empathy.

Most medical schools have an orientation week intended to introduce first-year students to different aspects of the school and for students to get to one another and the faculty, staff, and administration. Medical schools, including Boston University School of Medicine, Harvard School of Medicine and Johns Hopkins School of Medicine, integrate a racial equity workshop into that orientation week for students to learn about racial disparities in medicine, share stories about their experiences with race and get comfortable talking about racism.[11-13] Interventional studies show that these kinds of training and forums can help physicians better address racism by promoting effective dialogues on racism without requiring a significant time commitment.[14]

First-year clinical skills courses can also incorporate training on long-term, structural issues like racism. While learning history-taking, for example, medical students should be trained to screen for social factors by asking patients questions such as, "What do you do in your free time? Where do you shop for groceries? Do you feel safe in your neighborhood?" These were the kinds of questions that had helped Dr. L better understand Mercedes' lifestyle and environment and had led Dr. L to identify racism as a possible risk factor for Mercedes' health. These questions build trust and can open the door for further conversations about experiences with racism.

The recommendation for physicians to learn about and address racism in a clinical setting is just the beginning. A physician's role is to dig deeper into a patient's history and to connect patients with other individuals and organizations. This first step will initiate communication with an interdisciplinary team, including dieticians, social workers, and organizations such as support groups. Dieticians are the most obviously applicable to Mercedes' case.

However, an interdisciplinary team is necessary to tackle health problems that are related to systemic issues, such as racism. Social workers can help identify unsafe aspects of Mercedes' environment and relay this information to state organizations. Support groups can help Mercedes find community and provide safety in numbers. This multi-level cooperation can raise awareness about the effect of racism on health and mitigate racial disparities in social support and access to medical care.

On a larger scale, a physician's role is to use patient narratives to put a face to governmental issues. Mercedes' case highlights several relevant issues: housing discrimination, universal health care and federal funding for community health centers. Housing discrimination had forced Mercedes into health-harming conditions. Mercedes had postponed getting her physical and had to drive two hours that day because there was no other clinic nearby that accepted her insurance. Universal health care could have encouraged Mercedes to seek care earlier and more frequently. Similarly, increased funding for community health centers could help improve existing centers or open new centers in communities like Mercedes.'

Student groups, such as American Medical Association/Medical Student Section (AMA/MMS), can give medical students a platform to learn about and express their opinions on these issues. AMA/MMS is the largest organization of medical students in the United States. Many medical schools have a student group that manages the AMA/MMS chapter at the school.[15] AMA/MMS student and physician leaders teach newer medical students how to craft policy briefs. AMA/MMS offers the opportunity to attend policy-making conferences and vote on state and national issues.

Student groups, such as AMA/MMS, can teach physicians to identify racist policies and to be advocates for their patients on a larger scale. Along with facts and statistics, physicians can share their personal feelings upon having to send patients, such as Mercedes, back to health-harming conditions. On the frontlines of the obesity pandemic, physicians can counter those who blame the patients without acknowledging the broader factors at play. Addressing racism in this way can lead to hospital-, state- and national-level changes in progress towards health equity.

A Few Words on Health Disparity in the Asian American Community

October 19, 2020

Jasmine Lam
University of California Riverside School of Medicine
Class of 2023

AS STRESSED MEDICAL STUDENTS looking for an eventful destination to spend our spring break, my friend and I chose to take a trip to America's Big Apple, New York City. On a sunny day in NYC, I remember enjoying our morning cups of coffee and walking into a subway station when, suddenly, an older man shouted at us, "Take your corona and get out of my country!"

Having grown up in Hong Kong and Southern California where there are prominent Asian populations, I am fortunate to say I have never really experienced discriminatory events, especially none this direct. More than shocked, I was disheartened. Despite hindrances and inconsistencies in life, my ancestors never stopped pouring sweat to better this country we call home. Knowing that Asian American history is deeply intertwined with this country's development, it felt like our contributions did not matter when that man verbally attacked us. It felt like we were not welcome after all.

That got my friend and me, both Asian American medical students, thinking: *Are Asian Americans misrepresented and experiencing disparities within our health care system?*

Health disparity is a term that refers to the differences in medical resources and health outcomes experienced by social groups.[1] These groups consist of individuals of different gender, race, education, and socioeconomic status, to name a few. Despite significant research on health disparities, Asian Americans are among one of the least studied groups on this matter.

And why is that?

From our nation's history, there is a deeply rooted belief in the "model minority" myth.[2] This ideology stereotypes Asians to be more educated, financially stable and healthier compared to other minority groups. While this generalization might seem positive, it actually brings more harm than good. Such a social myth can undermine the struggles experienced by less fortunate Asian Americans. By generalizing the whole Asian American community using a few successful examples, Asian American folks in need are inevitably overlooked. In reality, certain Asian groups (Vietnamese, Hmong and Cambodians) have higher poverty rates than the national average.[3] In addition, suicide is ranked as a higher leading cause of death among Asian Americans than among other ethnic groups combined.[4]

Secondly, there is immense diversity within the Asian American community. In Asia alone, there are 49 countries with 23,000 different languages in use. Data also shows that about 70% of Asian Americans are foreign-born. In a clinical setting, the immense diversity of languages poses a language barrier to equal access to medical resources. According to research done by Dr. Grace Ma at Temple University, cancer is the leading cause of death in Asian patients. Yet, they have the most trouble understanding clinical instructions and the highest dissatisfaction rates in regards to their cancer care.[5]

Last but not least, many health providers are ill-equipped to discuss Eastern medicine with Asian patients. Growing up in an Asian household, I experienced Eastern medicine, such as tiger balm or herbal tea, like many people in our community. On several occasions, these products have worked wonders. Asian patients may resort to Eastern medicine and, in turn, oppose Western treatments. Since most Western physicians are unfamiliar with alternative medicine, such a preference can further pose a threat for disparity and miscommunication. As health care providers, we should educate ourselves on topics such as alternative medicine to better serve our patients from Asian American communities.

Asian Americans are not only a minority in number, but it is also undeniable that we are among the groups vulnerable to health disparities. As future educators and physicians, it is important for us to understand the factors that create health disparity in our system. Even seemingly positive stereotypes can cause us to overlook the diversity within a group and cause patients to suffer. Especially in a sensitive time when Asians are experiencing more xenophobia due to COVID-19, we should question societal beliefs and be cautious about our assumptions with all patients.

It's A Lot
July 9, 2020

Holly Ingram
East Carolina University Brody School of Medicine
Class of 2022

I agree that protesting is best done in peace,
But wasn't that tried by taking a knee?

Or hashtags that said Black Lives Matter,
And praying that change would come with the chatter.

Voices were raised, injustices shown,
So much was done without throwing a stone.

There were plenty of calls of action before,
Peaceful posts, rallies, discussions, and more.

Setting fires and looting wasn't first done,
It happened only after more shots with guns.

And it's not just violence that started the unrest,
It's finance, it's health, it's a community distressed.

It's role models, education, access to care,
It's life expectancy, jobs, and professional hair.

It's giving your children more 'normal' names,
It's Halloween costumes and make-believe games,

It's driving, jogging, and playing outside,
It's seeing a cop and wanting to hide.

It's voicing a concern and being dismissed,
It's the watchful eyes of an interracial kiss.

It's homeowning and judgement and proving yourself,
It's the disparities affecting mental health.

It's a visit at the hospital, then questioning your worth,
It's more mothers that have died while giving birth.

It's telling the truth, but them assuming you've lied,
It's needing painkillers but being denied.

It's assuming you're ignoring advice to take meds,
Instead of listening to what you have said.

It's being labeled as difficult and noncompliant,
It's avoiding the doctors since they seem unreliant.

It's searching for allies but fearing a foe,
It's remembering to go high when they go low.

It's dismissing the issues as a 'mix-up,'
It's being asked to explain what part is corrupt.

It's brushing it off if there was 'good intent,'
It's standing out at certain events.

It's being asked which country you're from,
Or saying your English is better than some.

It's carrying a burden that shouldn't be yours,
It's having to prove that you're not poor.

It's expecting you don't live in certain locations,
It's researching racism in spots for vacations.

It's systemic and endemic causing the trouble,
And some of us tend to just live in our bubble.

We all have bias, we all make assumptions,
With the best of intentions, we can still mis-function.

Acknowledging the issues is a good start,
Then working to change through policies and heart.

ADVOCACY: THIS IS OUR LANE

It's true that not everyone shown on the news,
Is representative of the same views.

Some are calling for their voice to be heard,
While others are crossing some lines that are blurred.

Some stand for change that may come about,
Some show their anger in hostile routes.

Try not to judge what's right or what's wrong,
But remember the inequities that have lasted so long.

Walk in their shoes and see through their eyes,
Remember the history and the previous cries.

Try not to accuse, or label, or blame,
And try not to forget all of the pain.

I agree that we shouldn't fight hate with hate,
But we shouldn't blame those who were put in this place.

Advocacy:
This Is Our Lane

•

refugees

> ADVOCACY: THIS IS OUR LANE

Providers, Not Puppets
July 17, 2020

Yasmine Suliman
University of California Riverside School of Medicine
Class of 2023

"IT FELT LIKE A FREEZER and all they gave us was a paper-thin blanket, almost like aluminum foil," Sameera explained, "We gathered all three of our blankets and wrapped them up into one for my daughter. My husband and I waited and prayed instead." Sameera was an Iraqi refugee who had recently arrived from Tijuana, Mexico. She fled violence from what seemed like every corner of the globe, starting with Iraq, then to Yemen, Brazil, Mexico, and now to a small, bare and cold cell somewhere in Southern California.

Sameera was the very first patient I had the honor of helping through the Medical Students for Immigrant Justice Asylum Clinic at University of California Riverside (UCR) School of Medicine. I sat by, furiously taking notes and holding back my tears, as she told the forensic psychiatrist her story. Any and every point that Sameera mentioned could prove to be helpful in her asylum case, so I made sure to cross every 't' and dot every 'i.' For millions of refugees and immigrants, the idea of moving to America seems like a solution, an opportunity to chase the "American Dream." Instead, I learned from Sameera that the U.S. government greets them with detention centers that separate families and treat detainees as subhuman.

As I started reading through asylum cases, I began to notice the clinical ramifications of detention centers nationwide. Their unethical and undignified treatment of immigrants was obvious, making headlines.[1] Despite this, detention centers still managed to gild their substandard care beneath the lie that comprehensive health care was their top priority. Private health care companies hired by Immigration and Customs Enforcement (ICE) asserted that they made "the best possible care decisions with the information that was available to them." [2]

However, the indefinite nature of detention, along with the toxic stress, lack of food and hygiene, and poor medical expertise available, proved to be more than detrimental for many immigrants locked up all over the country. Since 2003, more than 185 people have died within custody, mainly due to substandard medical attention, inadequate mental health care, the misuse of solitary confinement, and delayed emergency services.[3] Considering no changes have been made to the detention centers being utilized today, it becomes clear that regardless of the amount of medical care that ICE claims to provide, real care is not possible in such conditions.

For me personally, it is easy to blame structures like ICE and the Department of Homeland Security for their role in detention centers. However, the role of physicians and those recruited to serve within these systems is more complicated. On one hand, it is an obligation for physicians to treat detainees in need of medical and psychological services. On the other, it seems as though their cooperation allows these systems to continue without consequence. Physicians for Human Rights, a non-profit committed to advocating against human rights violations, refers to this concept as "dual loyalty."[4] It states that physicians hold responsibilities to their patients but also to the agencies that employ them.

In this case, dual loyalty creates an issue within detention centers for physicians who hold no clinical independence. Currently, health care providers are required to sign non-disclosure agreements, preventing them from reporting the true conditions of the facility they work within and the patients they are serving.[4] By abiding by these reporting rules, physicians are providing a service that could help justify expanding and recreating these detention centers in different locations, thereby putting more people at harm. Simultaneously, physicians' medical contributions are constantly underscored as detention centers continue to treat detainees inhumanely and limit the medical resources available to them. This puzzles me. A cycle of providing care to treat the downstream factors while ignoring the upstream determinants — was this all a physician could do?

Fortunately, the American Medical Association (AMA) principles of medical ethics are clear regarding issues like this, particularly in Article III: "A physician shall respect the law and also recognize a responsibility to seek changes in those requirements which are contrary to the best interests of the patient." Additionally, Article IX states, "A physician shall support access to medical care for all people."[5]

I was reminded of these principles when I read a piece by Dr. Samuel Slavin, an internist at the Massachusetts General Hospital.[6] He engaged with these principles himself when helping a patient who needed urgent chemotherapy but was on the brink of deportation. Throughout his piece, he weaves in the difficulties he faced as her provider, both in caring for her medical needs and in helping to ensure that her visa was extended so she could receive her treatments. Through Dr. Slavin's piece, I got to see how these two AMA principles can be applied. His commitment to people, and not systems or titles, exemplifies how to practice health care within a system that does not share similar ethical guidelines. He points out that "my training did not include prevention of death by deportation," and this reflection perfectly sums up the issues that medicine faces and will continue to face as long as immigrant detention centers are up and running.

Through stories like this, I realize that working within a broken system first requires acknowledgment. That does not mean being complicit or approving of the systemic conditions that created it but, rather, understanding our role and how we continue to perpetuate it. As health care providers, we cannot afford to be blissfully ignorant when so much is at stake. When public health measures have failed to make any real progress on health equity within the past 25 years, it becomes even more crucial that health care providers on the front lines are cognizant of the different public health crises that continue to haunt our communities.[7] We must be constantly aware of the role we play and seek solutions rather than uplift the very systems that create them. From there, we can begin to advocate for changes that will prioritize our patients and our shared principles.

Outside the walls of detention centers, I still think about how I can stay true to the oath I took when I began medical school. Every time I see a patient in clinic, I think about how our current health care policies can limit patient access to quality care. Whether it is a lack of health insurance coverage, limited access to affordable medication, or the compounded effects of unaddressed health disparities, every patient now presents to me as a conundrum of health care at large: how can I truly fulfill my duties as a provider if the system cannot support my patients? How can I expand my role as a physician to encompass sustainable changes for my patients? [8-10]

As of this moment, I do not have all of the answers. But I will always aim to promote the well being of my patients first and foremost. After all, medicine and advocacy have always been intertwined, and advocacy has given us the power and direction to help others. In Dr. Slavin's own words, "We are not quite so powerless when armed with the realization that meaningful advocacy can grow from the human connections at the core of our profession."

—

Author's note: This piece was inspired by Dr. Scott A. Allen, who truly exemplifies the meaning of medical advocacy and selflessness. I want to extend my deepest regards to you for all the work you have done and all the health care providers out there fighting for real change. Thank you.

Forced Hysterectomies in ICE Detention Centers: A Continuation of Our Country's Sordid History of Reproduction Control

November 2, 2020

Lucy Brown at Indiana University School of Medicine, Class of 2023
Meghana Kudrimoti at The Ohio State University College of Medicine, Class of 2023
Minji Kim at University of Miami School of Medicine, Class of 2023
Candise Johnson at University of Mississippi Medical Center, Class of 2021

THE RECENT BLACK LIVES MATTER movement, the COVID-19 pandemic and the ongoing fight for reproductive health access have created a burgeoning sentiment of unrest across the United States. This unrest reached a high point in September when nurse Dawn Wooten filed a formal complaint against Dr. Mahendra Amin, a Georgia physician working at an Immigration and Customs Enforcement (ICE) detention center, who she claims performed mass hysterectomies on detained immigrant women without consent.[1,2] While the country reacted in shock, the reality is that coerced sterilization against communities of color is not new. The United States has a shameful history of exploiting Black and brown women's bodies as part of a larger objective for population control rooted in white supremacy — and the medical field is partly to blame.[3]

Many members of the medical community have been instrumental in devising research projects, medical devices and clinical practices that have been used to forcefully sterilize women of color. In the 1960s, birth control researchers experimented on Puerto Rican women largely because they regarded overcrowding as the fundamental cause of poverty.[4] The researchers held deeply prejudiced beliefs that people living in poverty, including Puerto Ricans, should be extinguished from society in order to allow those deemed more "fit" to survive and reproduce.[5]

Rather than focusing efforts on improving socioeconomic status to address poverty, head biologist Gregory Pincus gave women birth control with significantly higher doses of hormones than the modern day oral contraception in his mission to develop the first form of oral contraception.[5] Despite women experiencing blood clots, nausea and even death, the experiment continued and the side effects were ignored. Women involved, many of whom were interested in avoiding pregnancy, did not know they were participating in a clinical trial or taking an experimental medication — only that the pills would prevent pregnancies.[5]

Even after the passage of laws ending segregation and defining ethical research practices, attempts to control childbearing and reduce overpopulation continued throughout modern day America. In the 1970s, Mexican women living in Los Angeles were systematically targeted and sterilized because physicians decided they were a leading cause of the overpopulation problem.[6] Dr. James Quilligan, an attending at Los Angeles County-USC Medical Center, was accused of privately admitting that, "[P]oor minority women in L.A. County were having too many babies ... it was a strain on society ... it was good that they be sterilized." Women lacking English proficiency were coerced into signing documents to which they did not consent or did not fully understand. Other women who received postpartum tubal ligations were in the midst of labor or anesthetized and never remembered signing the legal documents. Despite this breach of patient consent, in the 1978 class action lawsuit, *Madrigal v Quilligan*, the Judge ruled in favor of the County hospital.[7]

This case echoes what occurred in 1960 in Puerto Rico and allegedly happened this year in the ICE facilities.[2] While not always explicitly stated by the perpetrators, all of these tragedies reverberate the same, twisted logic: women of color are the root cause of overpopulation; therefore, it is morally acceptable to take away their bodily autonomy in order to stop them from reproducing. This reprehensible way of thinking has pervaded all levels of our society, and medical professionals are clearly not immune. Members of the medical community, including Dr. Amin, those involved in the Puerto Rico and Los Angeles sterilizations, and anyone who was complicit in such unfathomable acts, have ignored their ethical oath to "do no harm" and instead enabled forced sterilization to occur within the present day.

Reproductive justice is not just about having a choice to abstain from reproducing — it also encompasses the choice to be a parent, have multiple children, or none at all.[8] The continuation of reproduction control efforts is a disgrace to our country. American exceptionalism is clouded by our history of reproductive racism, and this history is clearly far from over. As a profession, the only way to serve justice and move forward is to address the damage we have done.

Therefore, we urge the medical community to take responsibility and hold Dr. Amin accountable by removing his medical license. We demand that the practice of forced sterilization be abolished to ensure that organizations, including ICE, never again allow this violation of basic human rights. Most importantly, we wish to acknowledge the women who endured unimaginable and unconsented pain and loss for the sake of medical sterilization. We urge that reparations be provided to these women and their families.

The Largest Humanitarian Catastrophe of Yemen
July 18, 2020

Leah Sarah Peer
Saint James School of Medicine
Class of 2022

CURRENTLY, 125 MILLION PEOPLE around the world are affected by humanitarian emergencies stemming from national conflicts, outbreaks of disease and natural disasters.[1] Centuries-old diseases like cholera continue to affect people due to lack of access to clean water for sanitation and hygiene. Medical supply shortages and damaged health care facilities put millions at risk of illness and death from preventable conditions.[2] Given our responsibility to aid humankind, health professionals should be at the forefront of confronting these humanitarian crises. After all, the Hippocratic Oath is the testament of a physician's duty to care for humanity. As medical students in training, we have made that oath and by doing so, hold ourselves accountable for the advocacy of the vulnerable.

I am calling for international solidarity and aid for Yemenis who are currently living in the worst conditions imaginable without clean water, food or shelter. Today in Yemen, there is war, an economic crisis, cholera outbreaks, the Chikungunya virus and COVID-19, all in the same country.[3-7] Even if Yemenis are able to flee from such conditions, European countries are unwilling to accommodate the influx of migrants.[8] As such, international support and collaboration are critical from a human rights perspective, where human beings must be respected before anything else and entitled to their own inherent rights as designated by the Universal Declaration of Human Rights (UDHR).[9] Without due intervention from developed countries, the Yemeni refugees are disadvantageously situated with their very futures threatened.

Among the migrants, there are children who, given the precarity and scarcity of resources, will face an inescapable reality of famine and plague. Thus, within the COVID-19 pandemic, there is a crisis of children's rights in many disease-stricken lands. Vast numbers are unable to access proper nutrition and are left forgotten. Children under the age of five aren't able to receive vaccinations in a timely fashion, and this may unfortunately result in a vaccination pandemic.[10] Besides this, the conflict in Yemen has affected education for the past five years, leaving almost 2 million children out of school.[11] The uncertainty, chaos and conflict in war-torn Yemen have robbed children of their futures by depriving them of education, and with the COVID-19 pandemic, chances of them going back to school or accessing resources to learn are slim.

Since the conflict began in Yemen, the country is also experiencing the largest food insecurity emergency in the world. Although the World Food Bank has sent barrels of donated food, Al-Jazeera and BBC report that these containers have been unable to reach civilians who are in great need.[12,13] This is due to the lack of available fuel coupled with damaged roads hindering the distribution of supplies.

Pregnant and breastfeeding women are hit the hardest by food insecurity, as they require the greatest dietary diversity of iron and folic acid.[14] The effects of malnutrition leave them with weak immune systems, and as such, they are deficient in the proper physiologic coping mechanisms needed to fight infections and colds. Furthermore, they have had to rely on untreated water supplies and unprotected wells for sustenance, placing themselves at risk of life-threatening illnesses.[15] Failing to assist these people is a shame for the international community.

The human rights violations mentioned above raise ethical concerns regarding the suffering and dignity of individuals dying in settings like Yemen.[16] While medical professionals strive to save lives, the practice of creating space for individuals to die in dignity is a fairly recent phenomenon and urges for a more humane approach to suffering. In a crisis as large as Yemen, physicians will face patients pleading with them to be cured as well as to have an end to their suffering. Medical training and literature unfortunately lack guidance for patients and for health professionals to be compassionate caregivers in theaters of humanitarian health care. As a result of this, physicians are ill-equipped to care for patients in low and middle-income countries requesting a less painful death.[17]

Despite insufficient training to be in these war zones, physicians may alleviate the suffering of Yemenis by simply providing water, putting up blinds to protect patients from the scorching sun or even acting as a friend to someone who is grievously injured. These small meaningful acts of compassion provide patients with respect and dignity, strengthen the physician-patient interaction and allow for human connection to blossom — just as they do in the United States.

Oftentimes, such measures are the difference between life and death. As medical students in training who are navigating our own trajectories to becoming physicians, such a crisis in Yemen teaches us to unequivocally uphold dignity, nurture compassion and, above all, to be human. If we fail to be compassionate or refuse to engage in simple acts of kindness, then by nature of being physicians we fail to live up to humanitarian values. Only when medical care is embedded with compassionate care will physicians fully grasp the concept of viewing patients as human beings and not as transmitters of disease in arenas of war and conflict.

There is a humanitarian emergency, the largest one the world has seen, in Yemen that stands at risk of exterminating people due to its crisis intensity. As citizens of the world, educating ourselves about these issues in war-torn countries is important. Our voices are the most powerful instruments for change and courageously demanding organizations to deliver services to Yemenis is now, more than ever, vital. The children of Yemen deserve to grow up in peace, not conflict. We have to strive to achieve a better future for them, and therefore international cooperation is necessary to prevent the loss of another 100,000 innocent lives. Ignorance and choosing to look the other way is simply not an option. Some of the humanitarian agencies striving to improve the situation in Yemen include non-governmental organizations such as Yemen Care, Save the Children and Saba Relief.[18-20] Everyone everywhere, regardless of their background or race, has the right to health, safety and education. As people, as professionals and as human beings, it is time to do better for humanity.

Aylan
July 19, 2020

Sharon Hsu
Albany Medical College
Class of 2022

A mourning sun cries as she tucks away
the night to uncover red and blue
slumps of fabric and skin on gritty sand below.
Brazen tides return to grasp at the shore,
but the boy lies still in darkened, sodden clothes.

They cling to what is pale and small,
he who was delivered into lullabies dissolving
screams and bullets into the haunted night,
forced to flee from a sea of violent red
to the turbulent sea of blue.

I think of him and grieve —
still.

—

Aylan Kurdi was a three-year-old Syrian boy of Kurdish descent who drowned on September 2, 2015 while trying to reach the Greek island of Kos by boat. Of his four-member family, only his father survived the journey. Published images of Aylan's body brought swift attention to the ongoing Syrian refugee crisis and Syrian Civil War, resulting in international calls for action.[1,2] More than 12.8 million Syrians have been driven out of their homes due to civil conflict, with over 6.7 million Syrians forced to flee the country and 6.1 million people who remain internally displaced.

Advocacy:
This Is Our Lane

•

public health

Doctors for Democracy: Why Being an Election Worker is Good Public Health

September 29, 2020

Rob Palmer
Yale School of Medicine
Class of 2021

MUCH OF THE CONVERSATION around voting in the 2020 primaries and general election has focused on the safety and feasibility of mail-in voting. But we must also protect the millions of Americans who vote in-person during these elections. While I have encouraged people to vote from home in the general election, millions of Americans will inevitably vote in-person.[1] Helping these people do so as safely as possible is a pertinent public health issue, one in which health care students and professionals can play a vital role by working at polls on Election Day.

Analysis of the primary elections suggests that having an adequate number of safely-run polling locations will protect the health of citizens and communities during the general election.[2] Research of the Wisconsin primary found that more COVID-19 cases occurred in regions that had the highest number of voters per polling location. One of the causes of increased voter turnout at a given polling location is the closure of nearby polling locations. For example, only 20 polling locations were open during the primary in Washington D.C., which normally has 143 polling locations.[3] Likewise, there were five polling locations in Milwaukee during the Wisconsin primary instead of the usual 180.[4]

A key reason for the closure of polling locations is that many elderly poll workers decided to protect their health rather than work.[5] The net effect of consolidating polling locations is a decrease in overall voter turnout with an increase in voter volume at the few remaining polling locations. The latter makes adhering to social distancing policies and hygienic practices more challenging.

Can you imagine asking your parents or grandparents to work the polls, knowing they'd likely interact with hundreds of people? It'd be unconscionable.

Rather than ask elderly poll workers to risk their health on Election Day, medical professionals and students can volunteer to work at polling locations. Health care professionals and students tend to be in a lower-risk population and are also well-versed in the public health practices critical to safely conducting an election during the pandemic (e.g., hand and mask hygiene, social distancing practices, etc.). Of course, health care students and professionals are neither immune to this virus nor devoid of conditions that increase one's risk of serious illness; it behooves everyone to comprehensively consider their risk before placing oneself in harm's way.

Even a modest volunteer effort among students and professionals could have a sizable impact on the safety and feasibility of in-person voting on Election Day. If only five students from every medical school in the country worked at a polling location, then we would add nearly 1,000 polling workers. And if a comparable number of nursing students from every nursing school also volunteered, then the total number would be nearly 10,000.

Given that there were more than 200,000 polling locations and 600,000 poll workers in the 2018 general election, adding 10,000 poll workers might prevent hundreds or thousands of polling locations from closing and consequently help over a million people vote.[6] Additionally, poll closures have often disproportionately affected communities of color and low-income communities, and thus preventing closures especially protects the rights of disenfranchised communities.[7]

If you are interested in being a poll worker, then go to Power the Polls to sign up. You'll be led through a quick and simple registration process specific to your area of residence. As the general election approaches, you will likely need to undergo mandatory training, though it varies by jurisdiction. You can learn more about the registration process and being a poll worker by visiting Power the Polls — and share it with anyone you think might be interested.

Good medical care encompasses both treating medical conditions and preventing them from arising. Indeed, as medical students, we're often taught to encourage patients to use seatbelts or to wear bike helmets. The scope of our care has only increased during the pandemic with recommendations for prudent hand hygiene and social distancing practices.

When it comes to voting in the upcoming general election, the logic is no different: as poll workers, we can use our medical expertise and health to help our patients and communities be as safe as possible when we exercise our constitutional right to vote. Let's rise to the occasion on Election Day to protect our patients and the integrity of our democracy.

We Have a Cost Crisis in Medicine. What Can Medical Students Do To Help?

October 17, 2020

Caleb Sokolowski
Wayne State University School of Medicine
Class of 2023

THERE IS A COST CRISIS in medicine: the health care industry accounts for about 18 percent of the GDP in the United States, and predictive models see this increasing in the coming years.[1] This is a problem for the country as a whole as an estimated 41% of working Americans have some level of medical debt.[2]

Because this is an election year, many say that a change in power will fix this problem, but no matter your political beliefs, a change in executive leadership is not enough.[3] In addition to going out to vote, medical students must do more. As students, we have the ability to influence both our patients and superiors. We have the power to change the next generation of medicine. Although there are many reasons for our bloated health care costs, medical students are in a unique position to influence how our health care system functions in the future.

40% of students did not understand the basic principles of the Affordable Care Act in 2010[4]

In medical school, we spend years learning about the vast intricacies of the human body but little time studying how the health care system works. This may be partly the fault of our institutions and accrediting bodies, who prioritize our knowledge of the Krebs cycle over how a patient will afford their insulin injections. However, we have an incredible opportunity to create change if we choose to learn beyond our institutional curriculum.

It is our responsibility to recognize that medicine is not just about cells and pathology but about human lives, and these lives are greatly influenced by the ability to access medical care for an affordable price. We must take the time to learn about the health care system that, pending massive structural changes, we will inherit. Books by physician-writers, including *An American Sickness* by Elizabeth Rosenthal, *The Price We Pay* by Marty Makary, and *The Long Fix* by Vivian S. Lee, all contain important takes on the issues and conversations in our health care system — including price transparency, the insurance industry, pharmacy benefit managers, and medicare-for-all. It is from these studies that we can grasp the reasons that brought our nation's health system to the place it is today, and start to foster creative solutions for a better tomorrow.

One-third of health care spending is waste[5]

During rotations, we are tasked with learning evidence-based practices for prescribing medications, ordering tests and undergoing procedures. This gives us a great opportunity to not only learn when procedures and tests are indicated but assist in the battle against unnecessary treatment strategies that don't follow current guidelines.

While I don't believe it is advantageous to question our preceptors for overtreating, as medical students we can still provide extra checks in the health care system. Instead of challenging, we can ask our attendings what the indications are for one treatment course over another. Something as simple as this could lead the physician to think about the various reasons they are prescribing such a treatment plan. This way, medical students are able to both learn and help curb some of the waste we see in the health care system.

18% of visits across the U.S. result in at least one surprise bill[6]

In addition to educating ourselves about health systems, medical students can work to educate our patients about their ability to demand transparency within the health care market. While there have been recent advances in health policy that improve transparency in medical billing, patients still need to have the knowledge to benefit from them.[7] Patients should be aware of their ability to ask what a procedure or office visit will cost them. They should not have to stand for surprise billing that can lead to years of paying off medical debt.

In addition to knowledge about transparency, patients should know of alternative models of care — including retail medicine and direct primary care. For example, the Surgery Center of Oklahoma City lists cash prices for procedures online so patients can shop for a fair price. Medical students can educate patients about these alternative models of care. This can empower patients to take control of how they are spending their health care dollars.

90% of the nation's 3.5 trillion in annual health care expenditures are for chronic disease[8]

As physicians in training, we often spend more time with our patients than our busy attendings. This gives us the opportunity to get to know our patients' lives and counsel them on the importance of prevention. Benjamin Franklin said many years ago that "an ounce of prevention is worth a pound of cure," yet this is often lost in our fast paced and overwhelming health care system.[8] Heart disease and stroke alone end up "costing our health care system $214 billion per year." [9] If we began to educate ourselves, and then our patients, about improving their lifestyle choices, we could eliminate a large share of the health care costs we see today.

The mean hospital cost per readmission can be higher than the initial hospitalization[10]

In a recent interview on Leading the Rounds Podcast, Dr. Brent James, who has been one of Modern Healthcare's "50 Most Influential Physician Executives," said that while some health care problems are unique to the U.S. health care system, failures in care implementation are not.[11] James says that if we were able to create quality systems that were up to par with the advances seen in medical science across the world, we would vastly improve both the cost and quality of our medical care.

Quality improvement projects can be as simple as increasing hand washing among health care workers, but they can drastically improve patient outcomes and cost. In the hospital, we should have our eyes open for simple fixes to the common problems we see around us.

I often hear from my preceptors that "the system is the problem" and there is nothing we can do about it. Contrary to this opinion, the system is only able to run if we as the next generation of physicians agree to be a part of it. Instead, we can and must demand change. We have more power than we know, and it is our responsibility to take advantage of this power because the physical and financial health of our patients depends on it.

IN-TRAINING: 2020 IN OUR WORDS

Medical Students Call to Flatten the Curve on Climate Change: Lessons from COVID-19

April 22, 2020

Sarah Hsu at Warren Alpert Medical School, Class of 2022
Natasha Sood at Pennsylvania State College of Medicine, Class of 2022
Harleen Marwah at GWU School of Medicine, Class of 2021
Ellen Townley at Creighton University School of Medicine, Class of 2023
Sarah Schear at UCSF School of Medicine, Class of 2021

WHILE AMERICANS GRAPPLE with the horrors of the COVID-19 pandemic, many ask how they can support their cherished communities and those risking their lives on the frontlines. Along with organizing PPE drives and providing mutual aid, there is something else we all can do to prevent our communities from facing crises like the one before us: *organize to address climate change.*

As medical students, we are embarking on a career to join our mentors and colleagues to protect health. While the toll of this pandemic has rendered it difficult to think about the climate crisis, now, more than ever we are reminded that our planet is sick. On this 50th anniversary of Earth Day, we must reflect on the lessons from COVID-19 and how they can equip us to tackle what the World Health Organization has called "the greatest threat to global health in the 21st century."[1] Honoring our oath to "first, do no harm," we must safeguard the health of our planet and communities. We implore Americans to vote for leaders who champion ambitious climate policies.

The Present: Lessons from the COVID-19 Pandemic

Despite warnings of an impending outbreak, we were unprepared for COVID-19, leaving our health system overwhelmed and patients vulnerable. Beyond our hospitals, COVID-19 is exposing unsightly health inequities.[2] Older adults, people with chronic conditions and communities of color suffer from higher rates of mortality from this virus.[3] Our current system of employer-based health insurance leaves those who are unemployed without health insurance. Simultaneously, lack of paid sick leave renders many low-wage essential workers unprotected. The added strain of these systemic inequities is stretching even our modern health system beyond capacity and perpetuating great and avoidable suffering.

The Future: Healing in a Time of Climate Change

Like COVID-19, climate change is a major global threat and health emergency. We have already seen increases in lethal heat waves, massive flooding in the Midwest and raging fires on the West Coast, all of which have harmed patients, health centers and economies.[4] Climate change is already increasing the global burden of disease, including increased hospitalizations for people with COPD, asthma and heart failure, and increased rates of birth defects, cancer and psychiatric disorders.[5] Additionally, due to human activity and climate factors, three out of every four new or emerging infectious diseases, like COVID-19, are zoonotic in origin, meaning they originate in animals and jump to humans.[6]

Like COVID-19, climate change will overwhelm already strained health systems and essential services. Researchers are increasingly worried about how first responders will continue to fight COVID-19 amidst predictions of flooding in 23 states by the end of May, a hyperactive hurricane season this summer and more wildfires in the West.[7] If we do not prepare, these compounding crises will debilitate our workforce, global supply chain and health care system. These situations, once unfathomable, feel all too real in the current pandemic.

Like COVID-19, climate change will exacerbate existing socioeconomic inequities. Without equal access to clean water, air, food, housing and health insurance, historically marginalized and vulnerable populations will bear the initial brunt of the health consequences of climate change. Extreme weather events will disrupt health care delivery, resulting in increased morbidity and mortality for people with acute and chronic illnesses.[8] Furthermore, 88% of the burden of climate change will fall on children as they are particularly susceptible to compromised environments.[9]

As we build a healthy future, these important consequences must be considered.

Call to Action

The nightmare of the COVID-19 pandemic offers a view of what climate change will impose on our future health system and communities if uncontrolled. As future doctors, on the 50th Anniversary of Earth Day we raise our voices in unison to draw attention to the urgency of the climate crisis.

We are moved by the solidarity of communities as they innovate and collaborate to tackle this pandemic. In the coming weeks and months, our government and society have the opportunity to recalibrate and rebuild for a more equitable, healthy future.

We urgently call on our elected officials to uphold their oath to protect the American people. We need more than adequate pandemic preparedness. We need a systematic transformation with the capacity to respond to the increasing number of health crises before us. Policies like universal health coverage, the Green New Deal and the Paris Agreement will protect our communities and health systems, paving the way for a future of economic prosperity and justice.

In honor of all those risking and adapting their lives during this pandemic, we urge our fellow Americans to vote for candidates who support climate action. We have the tools we need to combat the climate crisis and protect health. Now, we need the political will to use them.[10]

Together, let's vote to flatten the curve on climate change.[11]

References

Starting from Scratch: Building M1 Teamwork during the Pandemic

1. The Core Competencies for Entering Medical Students. AAMC Students, Applicants and Residents. https://students-residents.aamc.org/applying-medical-school/article/core-competencies/. Published September 8, 2017.
2. Hospital Care Team Members. Merck Manuals Consumer Version. https://www.merckmanuals.com/home/special-subjects/hospital-care/hospital-care-team-members. Published March 2018.
3. Medical Student Perspective: Teamwork: Your Best Ally in Clinical Rotations and Internship. American College of Physicians. https://www.acponline.org/membership/medical-students/acp-impact/archive/march-2017/medical-student-perspective-teamwork-your-best-ally-in-clinical-rotations-and-internship. Published March 2017.

STEP 1 in the Time of COVID

1. Coronavirus Update. Prometric. https://www.prometric.com/corona-virus-update. Published November 17, 2020.
2. Results of 2016 NRMP Program Director Survey. NRMP. https://www.nrmp.org/wp-content/uploads/2016/09/NRMP-2016-Program-Director-Survey.pdf. Published June 2016.
3. WHO Director-General's opening remarks at the media briefing on COVID-19. World Health Organization. https://www.who.int/dg/speeches/detail/who-director-general-s-opening-remarks-at-the-media-briefing-on-covid-19---11-march-2020. Published March 11, 2020.
4. Timeline of the Coronavirus Pandemic and U.S. Response. Just Security. https://www.justsecurity.org/69650/timeline-of-the-coronavirus-pandemic-and-u-s-response/. Published November 17, 2020.
5. Prometric announced that they will continue closures in the U.S. and Canada through May 31st with the exception of essential service programs. USMLE. https://twitter.com/TheUSMLE/status/1254785386368233479. Published April 27, 2020.
6. R/step1 - Prometric will randomly select and cancel 50 percent of all currently scheduled. Reddit, StepStudypartner. https://www.reddit.com/r/step1/comments/g64o5q/prometric_will_randomly_select_and_cancel_50/. Published April 22, 2020.
7. R/step1 - When do you think Prometric will ACTUALLY be open for us to take STEP? Reddit, PChoisauce. https://www.reddit.com/r/step1/comments/fzmy06/when_do_you_think_prometric_will_actually_be_open/. Published April 11, 2020.
8. R/step1 - You know the only thing worse than taking Step 1? Not taking Step 1. Reddit, Warbreaker. https://www.reddit.com/r/step1/comments/gb3cit/you_know_the_only_thing_worse_than_taking_step_1/. Published April 30, 2020.
9. R/step1 - Accidentally signed up for non-open test site May 1, now Prometric thinks I already took my test. Reddit, SadPanda. https://www.reddit.com/r/step1/comments/gbypr2/accidentally_signed_up_for_nonopen_test_site_may/. Published May 1, 2020.
10. R/step1 - "Who cares if COVID is going on... You should STILL be STUDYING." Reddit, RedditMedNoob. Published April 27, 2020.
11. 'I Have a Ph.D. in Not Having Money'. The New York Times. https://www.nytimes.com/2019/11/25/health/medical-school-cost-diversity.html. Published November 25, 2019.

REFERENCES

12. College Board Coronavirus (COVID-19) Updates. College Board. https://pages.collegeboard.org/collegeboard-covid-19-updates. Published April 30, 2020.
13. About the LSAT-Flex. The Law School Admission Council. https://www.lsac.org/update-coronavirus-and-lsat/lsat-flex.
14. FAQS: The MCAT exam and COVID-19. American Association of Medical Colleges. https://www.aamc.org/services/mcat-admissions-officers/faqs-mcat-exam-and-covid-19. Published November 4, 2020.
15. Amid COVID-19, make USMLE Step 1 pass/fail now. KevinMD.com. https://www.kevinmd.com/blog/2020/03/amid-covid-19-please-usmle-step-1-pass-fail-now.html. Published March 24, 2020.
16. R/medicalschool - [Serious] Change.org petition for the NBME to release consistent, weekly updates regarding board exam scheduling during COVID-19- please consider signing! Reddit, bullouspemphigoid. https://www.reddit.com/r/medicalschool/comments/g0sqwb/serious_changeorg_petition_for_the_nbme_to/. Published April 13, 2020.
17. USMLE Exploring Alternate Test Delivery Options. USMLE. https://covid.usmle.org/announcements/usmle-exploring-alternate-test-delivery-options/. Published April 27, 2020.
18. @AbouS_K. Let it be known that while med students have been told to adjust our expectations accordingly and have done so), nowhere has it been explicitly stated that the expectations of us will be adjusted accordingly; so yes, every new announcement is going to stress us out even more. https://twitter.com/AbouS_K/status/1254886433808093184. Published April 27, 2020.
19. How Med Students Are Stepping Up To Aid Coronavirus Efforts. Forbes. https://www.forbes.com/sites/briannegarrett/2020/04/09/how-med-students-are-stepping-up-to-aid-coronavirus-efforts/?sh=3d503acd7836. Published April 10, 2020.

Lessons from Quarantine

1. Covid in the U.S.: Latest Map and Case Count. The New York Times. https://www.nytimes.com/interactive/2020/us/coronavirus-us-cases.html?action=click. Published March 3, 2020.
2. 'You Have to Disobey': Protesters Gather to Defy Stay-at-Home Orders. The New York Times. https://www.nytimes.com/2020/04/16/us/coronavirus-rules-protests.html. Published April 16, 2020.

Should Medical Students Continue Clinical Rotations During the COVID-19 Pandemic?

1. How COVID-19 could disrupt clinical rotations for med school students. Marketplace. https://www.marketplace.org/2020/03/10/how-covid-19-could-disrupt-clinical-rotations-for-med-school-students/. Published March 10, 2020.
2. Medical Students and Patients with COVID-19: Education and Safety Considerations. AAMC. https://www.aamc.org/system/files/2020-03/news-coronavirus-medical-students-role-covid-19-031320.pdf. Published March 13, 2020.
3. "Are you worried about coronavirus?": A medical student perspective. in-Training. https://in-training.org/are-you-worried-about-coronavirus-a-medical-student-perspective-19336. Published March 13, 2020.
4. Medical students can help combat Covid-19. Don't send them home. STAT. https://www.statnews.com/2020/03/14/medical-students-can-help-combat-covid-19/. Published March 14, 2020.
5. Flattening a pandemic's curve: Why staying home now can save lives. NPR Shots. https://www.npr.org/sections/health-shots/2020/03/13/815502262/flattening-a-pandemics-curve-why-staying-home-now-can-save-lives. Published March 13, 2020.
6. Physicians' responsibilities in disaster response & preparedness (Opinion E-8.3).

AMA Code of Medical Ethics. https://www.ama-assn.org/delivering-care/ethics/physicians-responsibilities-disaster-response-preparedness.
7. Cassell EJ. The nature of suffering and the goals of medicine. NEJM. 1982;306(11):639-645. For a thorough account, see Bishop J. The Anticipatory Corpse: Medicine, Power, and the Care of the Dying. Notre Dame, IN: University of Notre Dame Press; 2011.
8. Association of American Medical Colleges. Table A-6: Age of applicants to U.S. medical schools at anticipated matriculation by sex and race/ethnicity, 2014-2015 through 2017-2018. https://www.aamc.org/system/files/d/1/321468-factstablea6.pdf. Published November 30, 2017.
9. Wu Z, et al. Characteristics of and important lessons from the Coronavirus Disease 2019 (COVID-19) outbreak in China: Summary of a report of 72314 cases from the Chinese Center for Disease Control and Prevention. JAMA. 2020;323(13):1239-1242.
10. The Novel Coronavirus Pneumonia Emergency Response Epidemiology Team. The epidemiological characteristics of an outbreak of 2019 Novel Coronavirus Diseases (COVID-19) — China, 2020. China CDC Weekly. 2020;2(8):113-122.
11. COVID-19 and fighting the pandemic of fear. in-House. https://in-housestaff.org/covid-19-and-fighting-the-pandemic-of-fear-1673. Published March 12, 2020.
12. New findings confirm predictions on physician shortage. AAMC. https://www.aamc.org/news-insights/press-releases/new-findings-confirm-predictions-physician-shortage. Published April 23, 2019.
13. What does the coronavirus mean for the U.S. health care system? Some simple math offers alarming answers. STAT. https://www.statnews.com/2020/03/10/simple-math-alarming-answers-covid-19/. Published March 10, 2020.
14. How much worse the coronavirus could get, in charts. The New York Times. https://www.nytimes.com/interactive/2020/03/13/opinion/coronavirus-trump-response.html. Published March 13, 2020.

The Role of Third-Year Medical Students During the COVID-19 Pandemic

1. Guidance on Medical Students' Participation in Direct In-person Patient Contact Activities. AAMC. https://www.aamc.org/media/43311/download. Published August 4, 2020.
2. Report of the WHO-China Joint Mission on Coronavirus Disease 2019 (COVID-19). World Health Organization. https://www.who.int/docs/default-source/coronaviruse/who-china-joint-mission-on-covid-19-final-report.pdf. Published February 16, 2020.
3. Why Covid-19 is worse than the flu, in one chart. Vox. https://www.vox.com/science-and-health/2020/3/18/21184992/coronavirus-covid-19-flu-comparison-chart. Published March 18, 2020.
4. Diamond Princess Covid-19 update: Confirmed cases rise to 705. Ship Technology. https://www.ship-technology.com/news/diamond-princess-coronavirus-covid-19-cases-705/. Published March 16, 2020.
5. Field Briefing: Diamond Princess COVID-19 Cases, 20 Feb Update. NIID. https://www.niid.go.jp/niid/en/2019-ncov-e/9417-covid-dp-fe-02.html. Published March 16, 2020.
6. Mizumoto K, et al. Estimating the asymptomatic proportion of coronavirus disease 2019 (COVID-19) cases on board the Diamond Princess cruise ship, Yokohama, Japan, 2020. Eurosurveillance. 2020;25(10):2000180.
7. Coronavirus Disease 2019 (COVID-19) - Transmission. Centers for Disease Control and Prevention. https://www.cdc.gov/coronavirus/2019-ncov/prevent-getting-sick/how-covid-spreads.html. Published March 15, 2020.
8. Wilson N, et al. Case-Fatality Risk Estimates for COVID-19 Calculated by Using a Lag Time for Fatality. Emerging Infectious Diseases. 2020;26(6).
9. American Hospital Capacity And Projected Need for COVID-19 Patient Care. Health Affairs Blog. https://www.healthaffairs.org/do/10.1377/hblog20200317.457910/full/. Published March 17, 2020.
10. Coronavirus Disease 2019 (COVID-19). Centers for Disease Control and Prevention.

REFERENCES

       https://www.cdc.gov/coronavirus/2019-ncov/hcp/ppe-strategy/face-masks.html. Published February 11, 2020.
11. COVID-19 puts unprecedented strain on US health system. Healthcare Dive. https://www.healthcaredive.com/news/covid-19-puts-unprecedented-strain-on-us-health-system/574275/. Published March 17, 2020.
12. @PeterAttiaMD. https://twitter.com/PeterAttiaMD/status/1240293938684018688. Published March 18, 2020.
13. COVID-19: Guidance for Triage of Non-Emergent Surgical Procedures. American College of Surgeons. https://www.facs.org/covid-19/clinical-guidance/triage. Published March 17, 2020.
14. Should Medical Students Continue Clinical Rotations During the COVID-19 Pandemic? in-Training. https://in-training.org/should-medical-students-continue-clinical-rotations-during-a-pandemic-19371. Published March 17, 2020.
15. Medical students can help combat Covid-19. Don't send them home. STAT. https://www.statnews.com/2020/03/14/medical-students-can-help-combat-covid-19/. Published March 14, 2020.
16. Coronavirus news – March 2020. Harvard T.H. Chan School of Public Health. https://www.hsph.harvard.edu/news/hsph-in-the-news/coronavirus-news-march-2020/. Published March 2020.
17. The White House Is Asking Millennials — Yes, You — to Stay Home to Stop Coronavirus. Vice. https://www.vice.com/en/article/bvg3wq/the-white-house-is-asking-millennials-yes-you-to-stay-home-to-stop-coronavirus. Published March 16, 2020.
18. Millennials say their parents refuse to take coronavirus seriously. Business Insider. https://www.businessinsider.com/millennials-say-parents-wont-take-coronavirus-precautions-2020-3. Published March 14, 2020.
19. These simulations show how to flatten the coronavirus growth curve. Washington Post. https://www.washingtonpost.com/graphics/2020/world/corona-simulator/. Published March 16, 2020.
20. Can medical students be the key to ending the Ebola epidemic? ASTMH. http://iamtropmed.org/blog/2019/12/16/can-medical-students-be-the-key-to-ending-the-ebola-epidemic. Published March 16, 2020.
21. @RedCross. https://twitter.com/RedCross/status/1240648456055730176. Published March 19, 2020.
22. Hollander JE, et al. Virtually Perfect? Telemedicine for Covid-19. NEJM. 2020;382(18):1679-1681.
23. Medical students in the US babysit for healthcare workers: Business Insider. https://www.businessinsider.com/medical-students-babysit-healthcare-workers-covid-19-coronavirus-2020-3. Published March 18, 2020.
24. Thousands of medical students are being fast-tracked into doctors to help fight the coronavirus. CNN. https://www.cnn.com/2020/03/19/europe/medical-students-coronavirus-intl/index.html. Published March 20, 2020.
25. Italy rushes new doctors into service as coronavirus deaths rise above 2,500. Reuters. https://www.reuters.com/article/us-health-coronavirus-italy-idUSKBN214245. Published March 17, 2020.
26. Government is considering using medical students to help in coronavirus outbreak. Pulse Today. https://www.pulsetoday.co.uk/news/coronavirus/government-is-considering-using-medical-students-to-help-in-coronavirus-outbreak/. Published March 5, 2020.
27. @NYGovCuomo. https://twitter.com/NYGovCuomo/status/1240798215663955968. Published March 20, 2020.
28. SAEM Disaster Medicine White Paper Subcomminee. Disaster Medicine: Current Assessment and Blueprint for the Future. Academic Emergency Medicine. 1995;2(12):1068-1075.

Medical Ethics in the Time of COVID-19: A Call for Critical Reflection

1. The Chinese doctor who tried to warn others about coronavirus. BBC News. https://www.bbc.com/news/world-asia-china-51364382. Published February 6, 2020.
2. Should Medical Students Continue Clinical Rotations During the COVID-19 Pandemic? in-Training. https://in-training.org/should-medical-students-continue-clinical-rotations-during-a-pandemic-19371. Published March 17, 2020.
3. Makary MA, et al. Medical error—the third leading cause of death in the US. BMJ. 2016; 353:i2139.
4. Schernhammer ES, et al. Suicide Rates Among Physicians: A Quantitative and Gender Assessment (Meta-Analysis). American Journal of Psychiatry. 2004;161(12):2295-2302.
5. Yaghmour NA, et al. Causes of Death of Residents in ACGME-Accredited Programs 2000 Through 2014. Academic Medicine. 2017;92(7):976-983.

COVID-19 Lockdowns: Are They Legal?

1. Jacobson v. Massachusetts, 197 U.S. 11 (1905). Justia Law. https://supreme.justia.com/cases/federal/us/197/11/.
2. Toward a Twenty-First Century Jacobson v. Massachusetts. Harvard Law Review. https://cdn.harvardlawreview.org/wp-content/uploads/pdfs/a_twenty-first-century_jacobson_v_massachusetts.pdf. Published May 1, 2008.
3. Illinois, New York, California, Nevada Tighten Restrictions to Fight Coronavirus. The Wall Street Journal. https://www.wsj.com/articles/coronavirus-deaths-surpass-10-000-globally-11584698319. Published March 20, 2020.
4. 'We Are All in Quarantine': 100% of NY Work Force Must Stay Home, Cuomo Puts State on Pause. NBC New York. https://www.nbcnewyork.com/news/coronavirus/nyc-hospitals-weeks-from-running-out-of-supplies-as-death-toll-soars/2335762/. Published March 22, 2020.
5. Institute of Medicine (US) Committee for the Study of the Future of Public Health. Summary of the Public Health System in the United States. The Future of Public Health. https://www.ncbi.nlm.nih.gov/books/NBK218212/. Published January 1988.
6. Tenth Amendment. Legal Information Institute. https://www.law.cornell.edu/constitution/tenth_amendment.
7. Commerce Clause. Legal Information Institute. https://www.law.cornell.edu/wex/commerce_clause.
8. Trump extends federal social distancing guidelines to April 30. CNN. https://www.cnn.com/2020/03/29/politics/trump-coronavirus-press-conference/index.html. Published March 30, 2020.
9. The Alarming Scope of the President's Emergency Powers. The Atlantic. https://www.theatlantic.com/magazine/archive/2019/01/presidential-emergency-powers/576418/. Published March 19, 2020.
10. A Guide to Emergency Powers and Their Use. Brennan Center for Justice. https://www.brennancenter.org/our-work/research-reports/guide-emergency-powers-and-their-use. Published December 5, 2018.
11. Deference to the Executive in the United States after September 11: Congress, the Courts, and the Office of Legal Counsel. Chicago Unbound. https://chicagounbound.uchicago.edu/cgi/viewcontent.cgi?article=2736&context=journal_articles. Published 2012.
12. Proclamation on Declaring a National Emergency Concerning the Novel Coronavirus Disease (COVID-19) Outbreak. The White House. https://www.whitehouse.gov/presidential-actions/proclamation-declaring-national-emergency-concerning-novel-coronavirus-disease-covid-19-outbreak/. Published March 13, 2020.
13. Here's a list of the 31 national emergencies that have been in effect for years. ABC News. https://abcnews.go.com/Politics/list-31-national-emergencies-effect-years/sto-

REFERENCES

ry?id=60294693. Published January 10, 2019.
14. Stafford Act Assistance for COVID-19 Pandemic. Steptoe & Johnson LLP. https://www.steptoe.com/en/news-publications/stafford-act-assistance-for-covid-19-pandemic.html. Published March 23, 2020.
15. Fact check: Can Trump use the Stafford Act to order a national, mandatory 2-week quarantine? USA Today. https://www.usatoday.com/story/news/factcheck/2020/03/19/fact-check-does-stafford-act-allow-trump-order-quarantine/2872743001/. Published March 21, 2020.

Precedented: Historical Guidance on Freedom and Health in the Age of COVID-19

1. British Reforms and Colonial Resistance, 1767-1772. The Library of Congress. https://www.loc.gov/classroom-materials/united-states-history-primary-source-timeline/american-revolution-1763-1783/british-reforms-1767-1772/.
2. Pounds, Police, and Patriots: How Colonial Reactions to British Quartering Transformed from 1756-1774. Wichita State University Libraries. https://journals.wichita.edu/index.php/ff/article/view/189/195. Published May 15, 2016.
3. British Reforms and Colonial Resistance, 1767-1772. The Library of Congress. https://www.loc.gov/classroom-materials/united-states-history-primary-source-timeline/american-revolution-1763-1783/british-reforms-1767-1772/.
4. Intolerable Acts. Encyclopædia Britannica. https://www.britannica.com/event/Intolerable-Acts.
5. Dunaway WF. The Virginia Conventions of the Revolution. The Virginia Law Register. 1904;10(7):567.
6. The Great Smallpox Epidemic. History Today. https://www.historytoday.com/archive/great-smallpox-epidemic. Published August 2003.
7. Boylston A. The Origins of Inoculation. Journal of the Royal Society of Medicine. 2012;105(7):309-313.
8. Burgdorf WHC, et al. Abigail Adams, Smallpox, and the Spirit of 1776. JAMA Dermatology. 2013;149(9):1067.
9. George Washington and the First Mass Military Inoculation. John W. Kluge Center at the Library of Congress. https://www.loc.gov/rr/scitech/GW&smallpoxinoculation.html. Published February 12, 2009.
10. Positive and Negative Liberty. Stanford Encyclopedia of Philosophy. https://plato.stanford.edu/entries/liberty-positive-negative/. Published August 2, 2016.
11. Barbarossa Hitler Stalin: War warnings Stalin ignored. BBC News. https://www.bbc.com/news/world-europe-13862135. Published June 21, 2011.
12. Anti-maskers explain themselves. Vox. https://www.vox.com/the-goods/2020/8/7/21357400/anti-mask-protest-rallies-donald-trump-covid-19. Published August 7, 2020.
13. Positive and Negative Liberty. Stanford Encyclopedia of Philosophy. https://plato.stanford.edu/entries/liberty-positive-negative/. Published August 2, 2016.

Cruel and Unusual Punishment: Incarceration in a Pandemic

1. See Coronavirus Restrictions and Mask Mandates for All 50 States. The New York Times. https://www.nytimes.com/interactive/2020/us/states-reopen-map-coronavirus.html. Published April 25, 2020.
2. WHO Director-General's opening remarks at the media briefing on COVID 19. World Health Organization. https://www.who.int/dg/speeches/detail/who-director-generals-opening-remarks-at-the-media-briefing-on-covid-19---11-march-2020. Published March 11, 2020.
3. Correctional Populations in the United States, 2016. Bureau of Justice Statistics. https://www.bjs.gov/content/pub/pdf/cpus16.pdf. Published April 2018.

4. Rubin R. The Challenge of Preventing COVID-19 Spread in Correctional Facilities. JAMA. 2020;323(18):1760-1761.
5. The gap between the number of blacks and whites in prison is shrinking. Pew Research Center. https://www.pewresearch.org/fact-tank/2019/04/30/shrinking-gap-between-number-of-blacks-and-whites-in-prison/. Published April 30, 2020.
6. World Prison Brief, United States of America. World Prison Brief. https://www.prisonstudies.org/country/united-states-america. Published 2018.
7. Mass Incarceration: The Whole Pie 2020. Prison Policy Initiative. https://www.prisonpolicy.org/reports/pie2020.html. Published March 24, 2020.
8. Wilper AP, et al. The Health and Health Care of US Prisoners: Results of a Nationwide Survey. Am J Public Health. 2011;99(4):666-672.
9. Prison Doctors, Nurses Say Health Care Behind Bars Has Ruptured. Hartford Courant. https://www.courant.com/news/connecticut/hc-news-prison-medical-crisis-20180917-story.html. Published September 18, 2018.
10. ACLU National Prison Project: Know Your Rights Medical, Dental and Mental Health Care. ACLU. https://www.aclu.org/sites/default/files/images/asset_upload_file690_25743.pdf. Published November 2005.
11. Montoya-Barthelemy AG, et al. COVID-19 and the Correctional Environment: The American Prison as a Focal Point for Public Health. Am J Prev Med. 2020;58(60):888-891.
12. No One Deserves to Die of Covid-19 in Jail. The New York Times. https://www.nytimes.com/2020/04/23/opinion/coronavirus-prisons.html. Published April 23, 2020.
13. Guidance for Correctional & Detention Facilities. CDC. https://www.cdc.gov/coronavirus/2019-ncov/community/correction-detention/guidance-correctional-detention.html. Published October 21, 2020.
14. Releasing prisoners during Covid-19 crisis makes good sense. CNN. https://www.cnn.com/2020/04/20/opinions/covid-19-prosecutors-prison-release-honig/index.html. Published April 20, 2020.
15. Prioritization of Home Confinement as Appropriate in Response to COVID-19 Pandemic. United States Department of Justice. https://www.justice.gov/file/1262731/download. Published March 26, 2020.
16. Sivashanker K, et al. Covid-19 and decarceration: Healthcare needs to lead the charge. BMJ Opinion. https://blogs.bmj.com/bmj/2020/04/29/covid-19-and-decarceration-healthcare-needs-to-lead-the-charge/. Published April 29, 2020.
17. Michigan Pathways Project Links Ex-Prisoners to Medical Services, Contributing to a Decline in Recidivism. Agency for Healthcare Research and Quality. https://innovations.ahrq.gov/profiles/michigan-pathways-project-links-ex-prisoners-medical-services-contributing-decline. Published August 27, 2014.
18. Brooker R, et al. Medical student experiences in prison health services and social cognitive career choice: a qualitative study. BMC Med Educ. 2018; 18:3.
19. Giftos J, et al. Medicine and mass incarceration: education and advocacy in the New York City jail system. AMA J Ethics. 2017;19(9):913-921.

496 Beds: Medical Students Call to Action

1. Coronavirus Disease 2019 (COVID-19). City of Philadelphia. https://www.phila.gov/programs/coronavirus-disease-2019-covid-19/. Published 2020.
2. As COVID-19 crisis deepens, out-of-state patients seek help at Philadelphia hospitals. The Philadelphia Inquirer. https://www.inquirer.com/health/coronavirus/coronavirus-covid19-philadelphia-hospitals-new-jersey-20200404.html. Published April 3, 2020.
3. With Hahnemann closed, its owner, Joel Freedman, lists Rittenhouse home for $3.5M. The Philadelphia Inquirer. https://www.inquirer.com/real-estate/home/joel-freedman-hahnemann-hospital-philadelphia-rittenhouse-home-for-sale-million-dol-

REFERENCES

lars-20191003.html. Published October 3, 2019.
4. Hahnemann workers say operations winding down; owners plan bankruptcy filing. WHYY. https://whyy.org/articles/hahnemann-workers-say-operations-are-winding-down-owners-plan-to-file-for-bankruptcy/. Published June 28, 2019.
5. Hahnemann University Hospital Closure FAQs for the Community. https://www.hahnemannhospital.com/SitePages/Closure%20FAQs%20for%20the%20Community.aspx. Accessed April 27, 2020.
6. City, state prepared to spend $15M to deal with Hahnemann fallout, request matching federal funds. Bizjournals.com. https://www.bizjournals.com/philadelphia/news/2019/07/15/city-state-15m-hahnemann-fallout.html. Published July 15, 2019.
7. Private Equity's Latest Scheme: Closing Urban Hospitals and Selling Off the Real Estate. The American Prospect. https://prospect.org/health/private-equity-s-latest-scheme-closing-urban-hospitals-selling-real-estate. Published July 11, 2019.
8. Penn and the 1918 Influenza Epidemic. University Archives and Records Center. https://archives.upenn.edu/exhibits/penn-history/flu. Published 2018.
9. The Flu of 1918. The Pennsylvania Gazette. https://www.upenn.edu/gazette/1198/lynch3.html. Published October 28, 1998.
10. Hahnemann Hospital Owner Joel Freedman Offers Shuttered Medical Center at a Fraction of Market Cost to Provide Assistance to Philadelphia in Event of Coronavirus Patient Surge. PRNewswire. https://www.prnewswire.com/news-releases/hahnemann-hospital-owner-joel-freedman-offers-shuttered-medical-center-at-a-fraction-of-market-cost-to-provide-assistance-to-philadelphia-in-event-of-coronavirus-patient-surge-301029400.html. Published March 24, 2020.
11. Temple's Liacouras Center, set to be Philly's coronavirus overflow site, almost didn't get built. Billy Penn. https://billypenn.com/2020/03/27/temples-liacouras-center-set-to-be-phillys-coronavirus-overflow-site-almost-didnt-get-built/. Published March 27, 2020.
12. Philadelphia Hospital to Stay Closed After Owner Requests Nearly $1 Million a Month. The New York Times. https://www.nytimes.com/2020/03/27/us/coronavirus-philadelphia-hahnemann-hospital.html. Published March 27, 2020.
13. Mission Critical To Save The Economy: Fed Goes Even Bigger With Massive Loan Help. NPR. https://www.npr.org/sections/coronavirus-live-updates/2020/04/09/830578037/fed-offers-2-3-trillion-in-loans-to-businesses-local-governments. Published April 9, 2020.
14. Can Philly use eminent domain to take over the closed Hahnemann hospital for coronavirus patients? The Philadelphia Inquirer. https://www.inquirer.com/health/coronavirus/hahnemann-hospital-coronavirus-philadelphia-eminent-domain-20200325.html. Published March 26, 2020.
15. As Hahnemann's patient count dwindles to single digits, Temple and Jefferson see uptick in patients. The Philadelphia Inquirer. https://www.inquirer.com/health/hahnemann-temple-patients-er-20190723.html. Published July 23, 2019.
16. Penn Med School Dean Says Philly's Coronavirus Crisis Won't Peak Until May. Philadelphia Magazine. https://www.phillymag.com/news/2020/03/27/penn-med-dean-coronavirus-peak/. Published March 27, 2020.
17. Fleeing coronavirus in NYC, pregnant women head to Philly area but struggle to find prenatal care. The Philadelphia Inquirer. https://www.inquirer.com/health/coronavirus/coronavirus-pregnant-new-york-brooklyn-media-penn-obstetrician-main-line-health-20200403.html. Published April 3, 2020.
18. This is the coronavirus math that has experts so worried: Running out of ventilators, hospital beds. The Washington Post. https://www.washingtonpost.com/health/2020/03/13/coronavirus-numbers-we-really-should-be-worried-about/. Published March 13, 2020.
19. Over 10 million Americans applied for unemployment benefits in March as economy collapsed. The Washington Post. https://www.washingtonpost.com/busi-

ness/2020/04/02/jobless-march-coronavirus/. Published April 2, 2020.
20. Doctors In Training Are Dying, And We Are Letting Them Down. Forbes. https://www.forbes.com/sites/jacquelyncorley/2020/04/05/doctors-in-training-are-dying-and-we-are-letting-them-down/. Published April 5, 2020.
21. Woman who died of COVID-19 refused to go to hospital, worried about bills, her son says. Pittsburgh Post-Gazette. https://www.post-gazette.com/local/region/2020/03/25/Woman-who-died-of-COVID-19-refused-to-go-to-hospital-worried-about-bills/stories/202003250139. Published March 25, 2020.
22. A teacher who showed coronavirus symptoms was charged $10,000 for her ER visit — and was never even tested for the disease. Business Insider. https://www.businessinsider.com/nyu-langone-er-charged-teacher-coronavirus-symptoms-10000-medical-bill-2020-3. Published March 11, 2020.
23. Coronavirus is keeping Philly medical students out of hospitals, but we are still contributing. The Philadelphia Inquirer. https://www.inquirer.com/health/coronavirus/coronavirus-covid19-penn-temple-jefferson-medical-students-20200329.html. Published March 29, 2020.

"I Can't Be Here Anymore"

1. Khawam E, et al. Treating acute anxiety in patients with COVID-19. Cleveland Clinic Journal of Medicine. 2020 May 14.
2. Cuthbertson BH, et al. Post-traumatic stress disorder after critical illness requiring general intensive care. Intensive Care Med. 2004;30(3):450-455.

Welcome to Medicine

1. Medical School Graduation Questionnaire. AAMC. https://www.aamc.org/system/files/2019-08/2019-gq-all-schools-summary-report.pdf. Published 2019.
2. Chung MP, et al. Exploring medical students' barriers to reporting mistreatment during clerkships: a qualitative study. Medical Education Online. 2018;23(1):1478170.

Unpacking the "Insult" of Being Called a Nurse as a Female Physician

1. 2020 FACTS: Enrollment, Graduates, and MD-PhD Data, Table B-3. AAMC. https://www.aamc.org/data-reports/students-residents/interactive-data/2020-facts-enrollment-graduates-and-md-phd-data. Published 2020.
2. Thanks for the Compliment, But I'm Not a Nurse. I'm a Doctor. Slate Magazine. https://slate.com/human-interest/2013/09/i-m-not-a-nurse-i-m-a-female-doctor-but-thanks-for-the-compliment.html. Published September 20, 2013.
3. This is the kind of sexism women who want to be doctors deal with in med school. The Washington Post. https://www.washingtonpost.com/posteverything/wp/2016/10/04/this-is-the-kind-of-sexism-women-who-want-to-be-doctors-deal-with-in-med-school/. Published October 4, 2016.
4. American Nursing: An Introduction to the Past. Penn Nursing. https://www.nursing.upenn.edu/nhhc/american-nursing-an-introduction-to-the-past/.
5. RN Programs - Registered Nurse. Registered Nursing. https://www.registerednursing.org/. Published August 16, 2020.
6. 'Forget About the Stigma': Male Nurses Explain Why Nursing Is a Job of the Future for Men. The New York Times. https://www.nytimes.com/interactive/2018/01/04/upshot/male-nurses.html?mtrref=undefined. Published January 4, 2018.
7. An Epidemic of Doctors Bullying Nurses Is Threatening Patient Health. Slate Magazine. https://slate.com/technology/2015/04/doctors-bully-nurses-hospital-mistreatment-is-a-danger-to-patient-health.html. Published April 29, 2015.
8. Top hospitals show bias for male nurse directors. Nursing Times. https://www.

nursingtimes.net/news/hospital/top-hospitals-show-bias-for-male-nurse-directors-17-08-2010/. Published August 17, 2010.
9. 2018 Nursing Salary Research Report. Nurse.com. http://mediakit.nurse.com/wp-content/uploads/2018/06/2018-Nurse.com-Salary-Research-Report.pdf. Published June 2018.
10. Structural Inequality and Diversity in Nursing. Minority Nurse. https://minoritynurse.com/structural-inequality-and-diversity-in-nursing/. Published October 6, 2015.

Becoming More Emotionally Intelligent, Adaptive Physician-Leaders

1. How to Protect Yourself & Others. Centers for Disease Control and Prevention. https://www.cdc.gov/coronavirus/2019-ncov/prevent-getting-sick/prevention.html. Accessed January 2, 2021.
2. Blumenthal D, et al. Covid-19 — Implications for the Health Care System. NEJM. 2020;383(15):1483-1488.
3. Monaghesh E, et al. The role of telehealth during COVID-19 outbreak: a systematic review based on current evidence. BMC Public Health. 2020;20(1):1193.
4. CARES Act Provider Relief Fund. U.S. Department of Health and Human Services. https://www.hhs.gov/coronavirus/cares-act-provider-relief-fund/index.html. Published December 21, 2020.
5. Medicare Telemedicine Health Care Provider Fact Sheet. Centers for Medicare and Medicaid Services. https://www.cms.gov/newsroom/fact-sheets/medicare-telemedicine-health-care-provider-fact-sheet. Accessed January 2, 2021.
6. Rubin R. COVID-19's Crushing Effects on Medical Practices, Some of Which Might Not Survive. JAMA. 2020;324(4):321–323.
7. LCME Accreditation. Association of American Medical Colleges. https://www.aamc.org/services/first-for-financial-aid-officers/lcme-accreditation. Accessed January 2, 2021.
8. ACGME Main Page. Accreditation Council for Graduate Medical Education. https://www.acgme.org/. Accessed January 2, 2021.
9. Clinical education starts to resume, haltingly, in many health-care fields. Inside Higher Ed. https://www.insidehighered.com/news/2020/06/25/clinical-education-starts-resume-haltingly-many-health-care-fields. Published June 25, 2020.
10. Jumreornvong O, et al. Telemedicine and Medical Education in the Age of COVID-19. Acad Med. 2020;95(12):1838-1843.
11. Block BL, et al. During COVID-19, Outpatient Advance Care Planning Is Imperative: We Need All Hands on Deck. J Am Geriatr Soc. 2020;68(7):1395-1397.
12. Coronavirus Vaccine Tracker. The New York Times. https://www.nytimes.com/interactive/2020/science/coronavirus-vaccine-tracker.html. Published June 10, 2020.
13. Ali S. Combatting Against Covid-19 & Misinformation: A Systematic Review. Human Arenas. 2020;1-16.
14. Desta TT, et al. Living with COVID-19-triggered pseudoscience and conspiracies. Int J Public Health. 2020;65(6):713-714.
15. Conti AA. Historical evolution of the concept of health in Western medicine. Acta Biomed. 2018;89(3):352-354.
16. Margalit AP, et al. A practical assessment of physician biopsychosocial performance. Med Teach. 2007;29(8):e219-e226.
17. Palmer RC, et al. Social Determinants of Health: Future Directions for Health Disparities Research. Am J Public Health. 2019;109(S1):S70-S71.
18. Rouble AN, et al. Integrating clinical medicine and population health: where to from here? Can J Public Health. 2019;110(6):801-804.
19. Birkhäuer J, et al. Trust in the health care professional and health outcome: A meta-analysis. PLoS One. 2017;12(2):e0170988.
20. Berry LL, et al. Patients' commitment to their primary physician and why it matters.

Ann Fam Med. 2008;6(1):6-13.
21. Laiteerapong N, et al. The pace of change in medical practice and health policy: collision or coexistence? J Gen Intern Med. 2015;30(6):848-852.
22. Heifetz RA, et al. The Practice of Adaptive Leadership: Tools and Tactics for Changing Your Organization and the World. Harvard Business Press; 2009.
23. Birks YF, et al. Emotional intelligence and patient-centered care. J R Soc Med. 2007;100(8):368-374.
24. Mayer JD, et al. Emotional intelligence meets traditional standards for an intelligence. Intell. 1999;27(4):267-298.
25. Goleman D. Emotional Intelligence. London: Bloomsbury; 2020.
26. Sánchez-Álvarez N, et al. A Meta-Analysis of the Relationship Between Emotional Intelligence and Academic Performance in Secondary Education: A Multi-Stream Comparison. Front Psychol. 2020;11.
27. Preece PF, et al. A classical IQ model of the stages of cognitive development. Intell. 1996;23(3):229-236.
28. Bradberry T, et al. Leadership 2.0. San Diego, CA: TalentSmart; 2012.
29. Schutte NS, et al. Connections between emotional intelligence and workplace flourishing. Pers Individ Dif. 2014;66:134-139.
30. Nightingale S, et al. The impact of emotional intelligence in health care professionals on caring behaviour towards patients in clinical and long-term care settings: Findings from an integrative review. Int J Nurs Stud. 2018;80:106-117.
31. Covey SR. The 7 Habits of Highly Effective People. New York: Free Press; 2013.
32. COVID-19 Social and Political Analyses. New Politics. https://newpol.org/covid-19-social-and-political-analyses/. Published July 13, 2020.
33. Törnberg P. Echo chambers and viral misinformation: Modeling fake news as complex contagion. PLoS One. 2018;13(9):e0203958.

Medical Students Do Not Owe You Their Trauma

1. Watkins J. Preventing a Covid-19 pandemic. BMJ. 2020;368.
2. Violent deaths of George Floyd, Breonna Taylor reflect a brutal American legacy. National Geographic. https://www.nationalgeographic.com/history/2020/06/history-of-lynching-violent-deaths-reflect-brutal-american-legacy/. Published June 3, 2020.
3. Why The Killing of George Floyd Sparked an American Uprising. Time. https://time.com/5847967/george-floyd-protests-trump/. Published June 4, 2020.
4. HHS Finalizes Rule on Section 1557 Protecting Civil Rights in Healthcare, Restoring the Rule of Law, and Relieving Americans of Billions in Excessive Costs. U.S. Department of Health and Human Services. https://www.hhs.gov/about/news/2020/06/12/hhs-finalizes-rule-section-1557-protecting-civil-rights-healthcare.html. Published June 12, 2020.
5. Match Communication Code of Conduct. National Resident Matching Program. https://www.nrmp.org/communication-code-of-conduct/. Published 2020.
6. Edwards F, et al. Risk of being killed by police use of force in the United States by age, race–ethnicity, and sex. Proc Natl Acad Sci. 2019;116(34):16793-16798.
7. Bryant-Davis T, et al. The Trauma Lens of Police Violence against Racial and Ethnic Minorities. J Soc Issues. 2017;73(4):852-871.
8. Markman JD, et al. Medical student mistreatment: understanding 'public humiliation.' Med Educ Online. 2019;24(1):1615367.
9. Singh T, et al. Abusive culture in medical education: Mentors must mend their ways. J Anaesthesiol Clin Pharmacol. 2018;34(2):145-147.
10. Doctor and Patient: The Bullying Culture of Medical School. The New York Times. https://well.blogs.nytimes.com/2012/08/09/the-bullying-culture-of-medical-school/. Published August 9, 2012.
11. Fleming AE, et al. Mistreatment of Medical Trainees: Time for a New Approach. JAMA

REFERENCES

Network Open. 2018;1(3):e180869.
12. Cook AF, et al. The prevalence of medical student mistreatment and its association with burnout. Acad Med. 2014;89(5):749-754.

Do I Belong Here?

1. Bravata DM, et al. Prevalence, predictors, and treatment of impostor syndrome: a systematic review. J Gen Intern Med. 2020;35:1252–1275.

A Defense of My Suicidal Peers

1. Plath S. Elm. Poetry Foundation. https://www.poetryfoundation.org/poems/49003/elm. Accessed December 2, 2020.
2. Wurtzel E. Prozac Nation: Young and Depressed in America. New York: HMH Books; 2014.
3. Physicians Experience Highest Suicide Rate of Any Profession. Medscape. https://www.medscape.com/viewarticle/896257. Published May 7, 2018.
4. Suicide. National Institute of Mental Health. https://www.nimh.nih.gov/health/statistics/suicide.shtml. Accessed December 2, 2020.
5. Fazel S, et al. Suicide. NEJM. 2020;382:266-274.
6. Bachmann S. Epidemiology of suicide and the psychiatric perspective. Int J Environ Res Public Health. 2018 Jul 6;15(7):1425.
7. Schwenk TL, et al. Depression, stigma, and suicidal ideation in medical students. JAMA. https://jamanetwork.com/journals/jama/fullarticle/186586. Published September 15, 2010.
8. Suicide prevention. World Health Organization. https://www.who.int/health-topics/suicide. Accessed December 2, 2020.
9. Suicide Prevention Resource Center. https://www.sprc.org/. Accessed December 2, 2020.

Soulful Medicine

1. Koenig HG. Religion and medicine I: historical background and reasons for separation. Int J Psychiatry Med. 2000; 30(4): 385-398.

Life as Chimera: When Life Combines with Itself

1. Wu J, et al. Interspecies Chimerism with Mammalian Pluripotent Stem Cells. Cell. 2017;168(3):473-486.e15.
2. Yamaguchi T, et al. Interspecies organogenesis generates autologous functional islets. Nature. 2017;542(7640):191-196.
3. Next Steps on Research Using Animal Embryos Containing Human Cells. National Institutes of Health, Office of Science Policy. https://osp.od.nih.gov/2016/08/04/next-steps-on-research-using-animal-embryos-containing-human-cells/. Published August 4, 2016.
4. Jonas H. Ethics and Biogenetic Art. Social Research. 2004;71(3):569-582.
5. Atlan H, et al. Does Life Exist? In: Selected Writings: On Self-Organization, Philosophy, Bioethics,and Judaism. 1st ed. New York: Fordham University Press; 2011:375-383.
6. Easterbrook C, et al. Porcine and bovine surgical products: Jewish, Muslim, and Hindu perspectives. Arch Surg. 2008;143(4):366-70.
7. Margulis L, et al. Origins of Sex: Three Billion Years of Genetic Recombination. New Haven, CT: Yale University Press; 1990:259.
8. Pascal B. Pascal's Pensées. New York: E. P. Dutton & Company, Inc.; 2006.

IN-TRAINING: 2020 IN OUR WORDS

Well It Happened: Step 1 Will Become Pass/Fail

1. Change to pass/fail score reporting for Step 1. United States Medical Licensing Exam. https://www.usmle.org/inCus/. Published February 12, 2020.
2. "Secretive Meeting" Threatens USMLE Reform, Critics Say. Medscape. https://www.medscape.com/viewarticle/914744_0. Published June 21, 2019.
3. Will the USMLE Conference Take Medical Students Seriously? How Board Examiners Should Score Step 1. in-House. https://in-housestaff.org/will-usmle-take-medical-students-seriously-1351. Published March 7, 2019.
4. Overtesting American doctors: The toxic pressure of board exams. BMJ Blogs. https://blogs.bmj.com/bmj/2019/02/12/overtesting-american-doctors-the-toxic-pressure-of-board-exams/. Published February 12, 2019.
5. Medical students are skipping class in droves — and making lectures increasingly obsolete. STAT. https://www.statnews.com/2018/08/14/medical-students-skipping-class/. Published August 14, 2018.
6. The Etiology of Application Fever. The Sheriff of Sodium. https://thesheriffofsodium.com/2019/03/02/the-etiology-of-application-fever/. Published March 2, 2019.
7. A Non-MBA's Guide to NBME Revenue in 9 Simple Charts. The Sheriff of Sodium. https://thesheriffofsodium.com/2019/02/01/a-non-mbas-guide-to-nbme-revenue-in-9-simple-charts/. Published February 1, 2019.
8. Dear NBME and FSMB, I watch HGTV more than Netflix: A Response to the Invited Commentary on USMLE Step 1. in-House. https://in-housestaff.org/dear-nbme-and-fsmb-i-watch-hgtv-more-than-netflix-a-response-to-the-invited-commentary-on-usmle-step-1-1274. Published December 30, 2018.
9. Chen DR, et al. Student Perspectives on the "Step 1 Climate" in Preclinical Medical Education. Acad Med. 2019;94(3):302-304.
10. Cheers and jeers as med school's Step 1 test becomes pass/fail. STAT. https://www.statnews.com/2020/02/14/cheers-and-jeers-as-med-schools-step-1-test-becomes-pass-fail/. Published February 14, 2020.
11. @SanjayPatelMD. The residency selection process is a daunting endeavor often assumed by faculty already bearing a ton of clinical (and other) responsibilities (thus with limited time). With hundreds of applicants/year, objective metrics are important. Pass/Fail is simply not granular enough IMO. https://twitter.com/SanjayPatelMD/status/1227701824121118720?s=20. Published February 12, 2020.
12. @VenkBellamkonda. Unpopular opinion: step 1 pass fail is a bad thing. With less objective differentiators, public biases show. Harvard gets in > Wisconsin. Man > woman. White > non white. Extrovert > introvert. Tall > short. Thin > obese. Christian > nonchristian #medtwitter #medstudenttwitter. https://twitter.com/VenkBellamkonda/status/1229566670248857600?s=20. Published February 17, 2020.
13. @jbcarmody. Since the announcement that Step 1 will go pass/fail, there's been a growing false narrative that USMLE scores allowed IMGs to compete on a level playing field with U.S. MDs for competitive residencies. Here is the uncomfortable truth - and what to do about it. (thread). https://twitter.com/jbcarmody/status/1228330688560144384. Published February 14, 2020.
14. @DoctorGao. This is a terrible decision and will disadvantage good students at lesser known schools. Of course the USMLE consulted no one about this. Another step in the dumbing down of our profession. https://twitter.com/DoctorGRao/status/1228107498030321664. Published February 13, 2020.
15. McGaghie WC, et al. Are United States Medical Licensing Exam Step 1 and 2 scores valid measures for postgraduate medical residency selection decisions? Acad Med. 2011;86(1):48-52.
16. USMLE Score Interpretation Guidelines. United States Medical Licensing Exam. https://www.usmle.org/pdfs/transcripts/USMLE_Step_Examination_Score_Interpretation_Guidelines.pdf. Published January 31, 2020.

REFERENCES

17. USMLE Step 1: Leveling the playing field – or perpetuating disadvantage? The Sheriff of Sodium. https://thesheriffofsodium.com/2019/01/13/usmle-step-1-leveling-the-playing-field-or-perpetuating-disadvantage/. Published January 13, 2019.
18. Results of the 2018 NRMP Program Director Survey, 2018. National Resident Matching Program. https://mk0nrmp3oyqui6wqfm.kinstacdn.com/wp-content/uploads/2018/07/NRMP-2018-Program-Director-Survey-for-WWW.pdf. Published July 2018.
19. @jbcarmody. Even with a scored USMLE Step 1, DOs and IMGs were not "beating out" U.S. MDs for competitive residency positions or specialties. Does this look like a level playing field? https://twitter.com/jbcarmody/status/1228330730205466625. Published February 14, 2020.
20. Khan M, et al. The Impact of Step 1 Scores on Medical Students' Residency Specialty Choice. Medical Science Educator. 2018;28:699-705.
21. USMLE Scores Should Not Dictate Specialty Choice. Medscape. https://www.medscape.com/viewarticle/919055. Published October 2, 2019.
22. Is Privilege the Real Prerequisite for Med School? Medscape. https://www.medscape.com/viewarticle/919999_2. Published October 23, 2019.
23. @vishal_khetpal. Most of the discussion, fundamentally, has focused on what this means for "us" – the people in medicine interacting closely with this exam (medical students, residency program directors, etc.). https://twitter.com/vishal_khetpal/status/1229160571049848839. Published February 16, 2020.
24. The dearth of black men in medicine is worrisome. Here's why. NBC News. https://www.nbcnews.com/health/health-news/why-dearth-black-men-medicine-worrisome-n885851. Published August 22, 2018.
25. @SonjaRaaum. The reaction to #USMLEPassFail has been across the board - and I have to say my own personal reaction has been as well. MS3 me, who scored a 197, feels relief Resident me, wishes I had let go of the shame earlier Course Director/APD me... well that's a bit more complicated. https://twitter.com/SonjaRaaum/status/1228182346840494080?s=20. Published February 13, 2020.
26. @theartof_gk. I'm not a physician, but my wife (@teaandreverie) is. I've watched her perform countless surgeries, counsel more patients than people I've met in a lifetime and work shifts that seem inhumanly possible. I've seen her bring home countless tokens of appreciation from people...(1/9). https://twitter.com/theartof_gk/status/1228360312082096128?s=20. Published February 14, 2020.
27. @AmolUtrankar. The transition to a pass-fail #Step1 should encourage med schools to: (1) Teach to understanding problem-based diagnostic frameworks over reciting facts. More @CPSolvers stuff, less Goljan or SketchyMed. [more] #MedEd #medtwitter. https://twitter.com/AmolUtrankar/status/1227922158527172609?s=20. Published February 13, 2020.
28. Lee AH, et al. I dream of Gini: Quantifying inequality in otolaryngology residency interviews. Laryngoscope. 2019;129(3):627-633.
29. Holistic Review. AAMC. https://www.aamc.org/services/member-capacity-building/holistic-review.
30. Hammoud MM, et al. Improving the Residency Application and Selection Process: An Optional Early Result Acceptance Program. JAMA. 2020;323(6):503-504.
31. Symbiosis: The USMLE, ERAS, and medical education. The Sheriff of Sodium. https://thesheriffofsodium.com/2019/03/03/symbiosis-the-usmle-eras-and-medical-education. Published March 3, 2019.

More Than Skin Deep: Underrepresentation of Brown and Black Skin in Medical Education

1. Bhopal R. Spectre of racism in health and health care: lessons from history and the United States. BMJ. 1998;316(7149):1970-1973.
2. How False Beliefs in Physical Racial Difference Still Live in Medicine Today. The New York Times. https://www.nytimes.com/interactive/2019/08/14/magazine/racial-differ-

ences-doctors.html, Published August 14, 2019.
3. Hoffman KM, et al. Racial bias in pain assessment and treatment recommendations, and false beliefs about biological differences between blacks and whites. PNAS. 2016;113(16):4296-4301.
4. Fourniquet SE, et al. Exposure to Dermatological Pathology on Skin of Color Increases Physician and Student Confidence in Diagnosing Pathology in Patients of Color. The FASEB Journal. 2019:606.18-606.18.
5. Fix AD, et al. Racial Differences in Reported Lyme Disease Incidence. American Journal of Epidemiology. 2000;152(8):756-759.
6. Ebede T, et al. Disparities in dermatology educational resources. J Am Acad Dermatol. 2006;55(4):687-690.
7. Akhiyat S, et al. Why dermatology is the second least diverse specialty in medicine: How did we get here? Clin Dermatol. 2020;38(3):310-315.
8. Petition: Medical schools must include BAME representation in clinical teaching. Change.org. https://www.change.org/p/gmc-medical-schools-must-include-bame-representation-in-clinical-teaching. Accessed November 29, 2020.
9. Nolen L. How Medical Education Is Missing the Bull's-eye. NEJM. 2020;382(26):2489-2491.
10. Mind the Gap: a handbook of clinical signs on black and brown skin. St. George's University of London. https://www.sgul.ac.uk/news/mind-the-gap-a-handbook-of-clinical-signs-on-black-and-brown-skin. Published June 18, 2020.
11. Fourniquet SE, et al. Exposure to Dermatological Pathology on Skin of Color Increases Physician and Student Confidence in Diagnosing Pathology in Patients of Color. The FASEB Journal. 2019:606.18-606.18.
12. Halder RM, et al. Ethnic skin disorders overview. J Am Acad Dermatol. 2003;48(6, Supplement):S143-S148.
13. Gutierrez C, et al. The History of Family Medicine and Its Impact in US Health Care Delivery. AAFP Foundation. https://www.aafpfoundation.org/content/dam/foundation/documents/who-we-are/cfhm/FMImpactGutierrezScheid.pdf.

You're Not a Bold, Knowledgeable Medical Student — You're Just White

1. Diversity in Medicine: Facts and Figures 2019. AAMC. https://www.aamc.org/data-reports/workforce/interactive-data/figure-18-percentage-all-active-physicians-race/ethnicity-2018.
2. Ross DA, et al. Differences in words used to describe racial and gender groups in Medical Student Performance Evaluations. PLoS One. 2017;12(8):e0181659.
3. Boatright D, et al. Racial Disparities in Medical Student Membership in the Alpha Omega Alpha Honor Society. JAMA Intern Med. 2017;177(5):659–665.
4. UCSF School of Medicine suspends affiliation with Alpha Omega Alpha Honor Society. UCSF School of Medicine. https://meded.ucsf.edu/news/ucsf-school-medicine-suspends-affiliation-alpha-omega-alpha-aoa-honor-society. Published June 5, 2020.
5. Youmans QR, et al. A Test of Diversity — What USMLE Pass/Fail Scoring Means for Medicine. NEJM. 2020;382(25):2393-2395.

Images of Violence Unravel Us — And Our Communities

1. Ahmmaud Arbery video was leaked by a lawyer who consulted with suspects. The New York Times. https://www.nytimes.com/2020/05/08/us/ahmaud-arbery-video-lawyer.html. Published May 8, 2020.
2. How George Floyd was killed in police custody. The New York Times. https://www.nytimes.com/2020/05/31/us/george-floyd-investigation.html. Published May 31, 2020.
3. Bruce B. The rise and fall of the Ku Klux Klan in Oregon during the 1920s. Voces Novae. 2019;11(2).

REFERENCES

This is Water: A Perspective on Race from a White Male

1. This Is Water: David Foster Wallace Commencement Speech. https://www.youtube.com/watch?v=8CrOL-ydFMI. Published May 19, 2013.
2. Redlining was banned 50 years ago. It's still hurting minorities today. The Washington Post. https://www.washingtonpost.com/news/wonk/wp/2018/03/28/redlining-was-banned-50-years-ago-its-still-hurting-minorities-today. Published March 28, 2018.
3. Infographic: Racial/Ethnic Disparities in Pregnancy-Related Deaths — United States, 2007–2016. CDC. https://www.cdc.gov/reproductivehealth/maternal-mortality/disparities-pregnancy-related-deaths/infographic.html. Published February 4, 2020.
4. Health Equity Considerations and Racial and Ethnic Minority Groups. CDC. https://www.cdc.gov/coronavirus/2019-ncov/community/health-equity/race-ethnicity.html. Published July 24, 2020.
5. CDC Health Disparities & Inequalities Report (CHDIR). CDC. https://www.cdc.gov/minorityhealth/CHDIReport.html. Published November 26, 2013.

Physicians' Role in Addressing Racism

1. Arroyo-Johnson C, et al. Obesity epidemiology worldwide. Gastroenterol Clin North Am. 2016 Dec;45(4):571-579.
2. Bombak A. Obesity, health at every size, and public health policy. Am J Public Health. 2014 Feb;104(2):60-67.
3. Byrd AS, et al. Racial disparities in obesity treatment. Curr Obes Rep. 2018;7(2):130-138.
4. People with certain medical conditions. Centers for Disease Control and Prevention. https://www.cdc.gov/coronavirus/2019-ncov/need-extra-precautions/people-with-medical-conditions.html. Accessed September 10, 2020.
5. A 'forgotten history' of how the U.S. government segregated America. National Public Radio. https://www.npr.org/2017/05/03/526655831/a-forgotten-history-of-how-the-u-s-government-segregated-america. Published May 3, 2017.
6. Redlining was banned 50 years ago. It's still hurting minorities today. The Washington Post. https://www.washingtonpost.com/news/wonk/wp/2018/03/28/redlining-was-banned-50-years-ago-its-still-hurting-minorities-today. Published March 28, 2018.
7. Jackson RJ, et al. Creating a healthy environment: The impact of the built environment on public health. Centers for Disease Control and Prevention. https://www.cdc.gov/healthyplaces/articles/Creating%20A%20Healthy%20Environment.pdf.
8. Health equity considerations and racial and ethnic minority groups. Centers for Disease Control and Prevention. https://www.cdc.gov/coronavirus/2019-ncov/community/health-equity/race-ethnicity.html. Accessed September 10, 2020.
9. Williams DR, et al. Understanding and addressing racial disparities in health care. Health Care Financ Rev. 2000;21(4):75-90.
10. Hall WJ, et al. Implicit Racial/Ethnic Bias Among Health Care Professionals and Its Influence on Health Care Outcomes: A Systematic Review. Am J Public Health. 2015;105(12):60-76.
11. Diversity & inclusion. Boston University. https://www.bu.edu/diversity. Accessed September 10, 2020.
12. Diversity and inclusion. Harvard Medical School. https://hms.harvard.edu/about-hms/campus-culture/diversity-inclusion. Accessed September 10, 2020.
13. Office of diversity, inclusion, and health equity. Johns Hopkins Medicine. https://www.hopkinsmedicine.org/diversity. Accessed September 10, 2020.
14. Hardeman RR, et al. Developing a medical school curriculum on racism: multidisciplinary, multiracial conversations informed by public health critical race praxis (PHCRP). Ethn Dis. 2018;28(1):271-278.
15. Medical student section (MSS). American Medical Association. https://www.ama-assn.org/member-groups-sections/medical-students. Accessed September 10, 2020.

A Few Words on Health Disparity in the Asian American Community

1. Health Disparities Among Youth. Centers for Disease Control and Prevention. https://www.cdc.gov/healthyyouth/disparities/index.htm. Published November 24, 2020.
2. What Is the Model Minority Myth? Tolerance. https://www.tolerance.org/magazine/what-is-the-model-minority-myth. Published March 21, 2019.
3. Southeast Asian Americans at a Glance: Statistical Profile 2010. SEARAC. https://www.searac.org/demographics/southeast-asian-americans-glance-statistical-profile-2010/. Published April 16, 2018.
4. Suicide Among Asian Americans. Asian American Psychological Association. https://www.apa.org/pi/oema/resources/ethnicity-health/asian-american/suicide-fact-sheet.pdf. Published May 2012.
5. NIMHD Grantee Talks Asian Health Disparity Research. National Institute of Minority Health and Health Disparities. https://www.nimhd.nih.gov/news-events/features/training-workforce-dev/center-asian-health.html. Accessed August 6, 2020.

Providers, Not Puppets

1. What Is Happening at Migrant Detention Centers? What to Know. Time. https://time.com/5623148/migrant-detention-centers-conditions. Published July 12, 2019.
2. Medical care in immigrant detention centers under fire. CNN. https://www.cnn.com/2019/10/04/us/immigrant-medical-care-wellpath-invs/index.html. Published October 4, 2019.
3. Medical Neglect. Freedom for Immigrants. https://www.freedomforimmigrants.org/medical-neglect. Accessed December 2, 2020.
4. Spiegel P, et al. Can Physicians Work in US Immigration Detention Facilities While Upholding Their Hippocratic Oath? JAMA. 2019;322(15):1445-1446.
5. AMA Principles of Medical Ethics. American Medical Association. https://www.ama-assn.org/about/publications-newsletters/ama-principles-medical-ethics. Accessed December 2, 2020.
6. Slavin SD. Doctoring and Deportation. JAMA. 2020;323(2):119-120.
7. Zimmerman FJ, et al. Trends in Health Equity in the United States by Race/Ethnicity, Sex, and Income, 1993-2017. JAMA Netw Open. 2019;2(6):e196386.
8. 87M Adults Were Uninsured or Underinsured in 2018, Survey Says. U.S. News & World Report. https://www.usnews.com/news/healthiest-communities/articles/2019-02-07/lack-of-health-insurance-coverage-leads-people-to-avoid-seeking-care. Published February 7, 2019.
9. Here's why many prescription drugs in the US cost so much—and it's not innovation or improvement. CNBC. https://www.cnbc.com/2019/01/10/why-prescription-drugs-in-the-us-cost-so-much.html. Published January 14, 2019.
10. Baciu A, et al. The State of Health Disparities in the United States. Communities in Action: Pathways to Health Equity. https://www.ncbi.nlm.nih.gov/books/NBK425844/. Published January 11, 2017.

REFERENCES

Forced Hysterectomies in ICE Detention Centers: A Continuation of Our Country's Sordid History of Reproduction Control

1. Lawyers allege abuse of migrant women by gynecologist for Georgia ICE detention center. NBC News. https://www.nbcnews.com/news/latino/nurse-questions-medical-care-operations-detainees-immigration-jail-georgia-n1240110. Published September 17, 2020.
2. Lack of Medical Care, Unsafe Work Practices, and Absence of Adequate Protection Against COVID-19 for Detained Immigrants and Employees Alike at the Irwin County Detention Center. Border Resource. https://borderresource.org/lack-of-medical-care-unsafe-work-practices-and-absence-of-adequate-protection-against-covid-19-for-detained-immigrants-and-employees-alike-at-the-irwin-county-detention-center. Published September 14, 2020.
3. Ross LJ. The Color of Choice. In: Color of Violence: the INCITE! Anthology. Durham, London: Duke University Press; 2016.
4. Guinea pigs or pioneers? How Puerto Rican women were used to test the birth control pill. The Washington Post. https://www.washingtonpost.com/news/retropolis/wp/2017/05/09/guinea-pigs-or-pioneers-how-puerto-rican-women-were-used-to-test-the-birth-control-pill/. Published June 12, 2020.
5. The First Birth Control Pill Used Puerto Rican Women as Guinea Pigs. History.com. https://www.history.com/news/birth-control-pill-history-puerto-rico-enovid. Published May 9, 2018.
6. Forced Sterilizations: A Long and Sordid History. ACLU of Southern Caifornia. https://www.aclusocal.org/en/news/forced-sterilizations-long-and-sordid-history. Published November 2, 2016.
7. 'No Más Bebés' revives 1975 forced-sterilization lawsuit in L.A. Los Angeles Times. http://www.latimes.com/entertainment/movies/la-et-laff-no-mas-bebes-20150612-story.html. Published June 12, 2015.
8. SisterSong, Inc. Reproductive Justice. Sister Song. https://www.sistersong.net/reproductive-justice. Accessed November 30, 2020.

The Largest Humanitarian Catastrophe of Yemen

1. Highlighting health in humanitarian emergencies. World Health Organization. https://www.who.int/hac/events/whscommentaries/en/. Published May 26, 2016.
2. Shortage of personal protective equipment endangering health workers worldwide. WHO. https://www.who.int/news-room/detail/03-03-2020-shortage-of-personal-protective-equipment-endangering-health-workers-worldwide. Published March 3, 2020.
3. Yemen crisis: Why is there a war? BBC News. https://www.bbc.com/news/world-middle-east-29319423. Published June 19, 2020.
4. Beyond the war: The deep roots of Yemen's economic crisis. The New Arab. https://english.alaraby.co.uk/english/indepth/2019/2/8/the-deep-roots-of-yemens-economic-crisis. Published February 8, 2019.
5. Largest cholera outbreak on record continues. Outbreak Observatory. https://www.outbreakobservatory.org/outbreakthursday-1/1/16/2020/large-cholera-outbreak-on-record-continues-in-yemen. Published January 16, 2020.
6. Yemen: Epidemics kill over 600 people in Aden. Anadolu Agency. https://www.aa.com.tr/en/latest-on-coronavirus-outbreak/yemen-epidemics-kill-over-600-people-in-aden/1840245. Published May 14, 2020.
7. Coronavirus: Five reasons why it is so bad in Yemen. BBC News. https://www.bbc.com/news/world-middle-east-53106164. Published June 20, 2020.
8. Europe's Failure to Uphold Refugee Rights During COVID-19. https://ilg2.org/2020/05/10/europes-failure-to-uphold-refugee-rights-during-covid-19/. Published May 10, 2020.

9. Universal Declaration of Human Rights. United Nations. https://www.un.org/en/universal-declaration-human-rights/index.html. Accessed January 6, 2021.
10. 80 million children can't get vaccines because of the coronavirus pandemic: WHO. Global News. https://globalnews.ca/news/6973926/routine-vaccination-coronavirus-report/. Published May 22, 2020.
11. As school year starts in Yemen, 2 million children are out of school and another 3.7 million are at risk of dropping out. UNICEF. https://www.unicef.org/press-releases/school-year-starts-yemen-2-million-children-are-out-school-and-another-37-million. Published January 4, 2021.
12. UN: Yemen's Houthi rebels blocking food for tens of thousands. Al Jazeera. https://www.aljazeera.com/news/2019/06/yemen-houthi-rebels-block-food-tens-thousands-190625072632971.html. Published June 25, 2019.
13. Yemen crisis: UN partially suspends food aid. BBC News. https://www.bbc.com/news/world-middle-east-48716258. Published June 21, 2019.
14. As crisis escalates in Yemen, pregnant women need essential care. UNFPA. https://www.unfpa.org/fr/node/15181. Published April 16, 2016.
15. Water, Sanitation and Hygiene. UNICEF Yemen. https://www.unicef.org/yemen/water-sanitation-and-hygiene. Published June 16, 2020.
16. Hunt M, et al. Moral experiences of humanitarian health professionals caring for patients who are dying or likely to die in a humanitarian crisis. Journal of International Humanitarian Action. 2018;3(12).
17. Hunt M, et al. Moral experiences of humanitarian health professionals caring for patients who are dying or likely to die in a humanitarian crisis. Journal of International Humanitarian Action. 2018;3(12).
18. CARE's Humanitarian Work in Yemen. CARE. https://www.care.org/country/yemen. Published May 27, 2020.
19. Help Children in Yemen. Save the Children. https://www.savethechildren.org/us/what-we-do/where-we-work/greater-middle-east-eurasia/yemen. Accessed January 6, 2021.
20. Yemen, Humanity and Hope. Saba Relief. https://www.sabarelief.org/. Published December 18, 2020.

Aylan

1. Troubling image of drowned boy captivates, horrifies. Reuters. https://www.reuters.com/article/us-europe-migrants-turkey/troubling-image-of-drowned-boy-captivates-horrifies-idUSKCN0R20IJ20150902. Published September 2, 2015.
2. Syria Refugee Crisis Explained. USA for UNHCR. https://www.unrefugees.org/news/syria-refugee-crisis-explained/. Published June 30, 2020.

Doctors for Democracy: Why Being an Election Worker is Good Public Health

1. Doctors and Democracy: Why Vote-By-Mail is Good Public Health. The Health Care Blog. https://thehealthcareblog.com/blog/2020/07/13/doctors-and-democracy-why-vote-by-mail-is-good-public-health/. Published July 13, 2020.
2. Cotti CD, et al. The Relationship between In-Person Voting, Consolidated Polling Locations, and Absentee Voting on COVID-19: Evidence from the Wisconsin Primary. SSRN. https://papers.ssrn.com/sol3/papers.cfm?abstract_id=3597233. Published May 11, 2020.
3. Primary voters in 8 states and D.C. faced some confusion, long lines and poor social distancing. The Washington Post. https://www.washingtonpost.com/politics/in-pennsylvania-officials-prepare-for-coronavirus-civil-unrest-to-disrupt-tuesday-primary/2020/06/02/96a55c40-a4be-11ea-b619-3f9133bbb482_story.html. Published June 3, 2020.

REFERENCES

4. Why did Milwaukee have just 5 polling places? Aldermen want answers. Milwaukee Journal Sentinel. https://www.jsonline.com/story/news/politics/elections/2020/04/10/coronavirus-milwaukee-aldermen-want-answers-polling-places-primary-election/5127577002/. Published April 10, 2020.
5. Studies and Reports: U.S. Election Assistance Commission. https://www.eac.gov/research-and-data/studies-and-reports. Published June 27, 2019.
6. Studies and Reports: U.S. Election Assistance Commission. https://www.eac.gov/research-and-data/studies-and-reports. Published June 27, 2019.
7. Morris K, et al. Voting in a Pandemic: COVID-19 and Primary Turnout in Milwaukee, Wisconsin. SSRN. https://papers.ssrn.com/sol3/papers.cfm?abstract_id=3634058. Published June 25, 2020.

We Have a Cost Crisis in Medicine, What Can Medical Students Do To Help?

1. U.S. health care expenditure as a percentage of GDP 1960-2020. Statista. https://www.statista.com/statistics/184968/us-health-expenditure-as-percent-of-gdp-since-1960. Published June 8, 2020.
2. Survey: 79 Million Americans Have Problems with Medical Bills or Debt. The Commonwealth Fund. https://www.commonwealthfund.org/publications/newsletter-article/survey-79-million-americans-have-problems-medical-bills-or-debt. Accessed October 16, 2020.
3. Joe Biden's Obamacare Opportunity. Vox. https://www.vox.com/policy-and-politics/2020/8/20/21372511/joe-biden-obamacare-health-care-plan. Published August 20, 2020.
4. Medical Students Lack of Knowledge of Healthcare Overhaul. Reuters Health. https://www.reuters.com/article/us-med-students-lack-knowledge-of-health/medical-students-lack-knowledge-of-healthcare-overhaul-idUSBRE88O1BV20120925. Published September 25, 2012.
5. Reducing Waste in Health Care. Health Affairs. https://www.healthaffairs.org/do/10.1377/hpb20121213.959735/full/. Published December 13, 2012.
6. Pollitz K, et al. US Statistics on Surprise Medical Billing. JAMA. 2020;323(6):498.
7. Executive Order on Improving Price and Quality Transparency in American Healthcare to Put Patients First. The White House. https://www.whitehouse.gov/presidential-actions/executive-order-improving-price-quality-transparency-american-healthcare-put-patients-first/. Published June 24, 2019.
8. Benjamin Franklin Quotable Quote. Goodreads. https://www.goodreads.com/quotes/247269-an-ounce-of-prevention-is-worth-a-pound-of-cure. Accessed October 16, 2020.
9. Health and Economic Cost of Chronic Diseases. Centers for Disease Control and Prevention. https://www.cdc.gov/chronicdisease/about/costs/index.htm. Published November 17, 2020.
10. Spyropoulos AC, et al. Direct Medical Costs of Venous Thromboembolism and Subsequent Hospital Readmission Rates: An Administrative Claims Analysis From 30 Managed Care Organizations. J Manag Care Spec Pharm, 2007 Jul;13(6):475-486.
11. 50 Most Influential Physician Executives, 2013. Modern Healthcare. https://www.modernhealthcare.com/awards/50-most-influential-physician-executives-2013. Accessed October 16, 2020.

Medical Students Call to Flatten the Curve on Climate Change: Lessons from COVID-19

1. WHO calls for urgent action to protect health from climate change. World Health Organization. http://www.who.int/globalchange/global-campaign/cop21/en/. Accessed November 27, 2020.
2. COVID-19: The painful price of ignoring health inequities. BMJ Blogs. https://blogs.bmj.com/bmj/2020/03/18/covid-19-the-painful-price-of-ignoring-health-inequities/. Published March 18, 2020.
3. Health care disparities in the age of coronavirus. Harvard Gazette. https://news.harvard.edu/gazette/story/2020/04/health-care-disparities-in-the-age-of-coronavirus/. Published April 14, 2020.
4. Climate Change Is Accelerating, Bringing World 'Dangerously Close' to Irreversible Change. The New York Times. https://www.nytimes.com/2019/12/04/climate/climate-change-acceleration.html. Published December 4, 2019.
5. Watts N. The 2019 report of The Lancet Countdown on health and climate change: ensuring that the health of a child born today is not defined by a changing climate. The Lancet. 2019;394(10211):1836-1878.
6. Zoonotic Diseases. Centers for Disease Control. https://www.cdc.gov/onehealth/basics/zoonotic-diseases.html. Published February 19, 2020.
7. Stressed by Coronavirus, First Responders Prep for a Dangerous Summer. Vanity Fair. https://www.vanityfair.com/news/2020/04/stressed-by-coronavirus-first-responders-prep-for-a-dangerous-summer. Published April 12, 2020.
8. Curtis S, et al. Impact of extreme weather events and climate change for health and social care systems. Environ Health. 2017;16(1):128.
9. Zhang Y, et al. Climate change and disability-adjusted life years. J Environ Health. 2007;70(3):32-36.
10. Project Drawdown. https://drawdown.org/. Accessed November 27, 2020.
11. Register to vote. Vote.gov. https://vote.gov/. Accessed November 27, 2020.

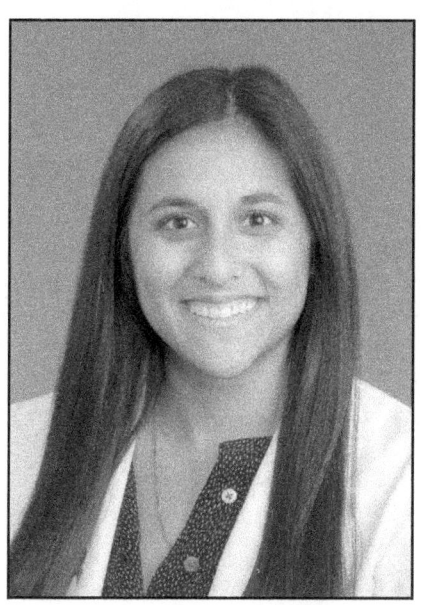 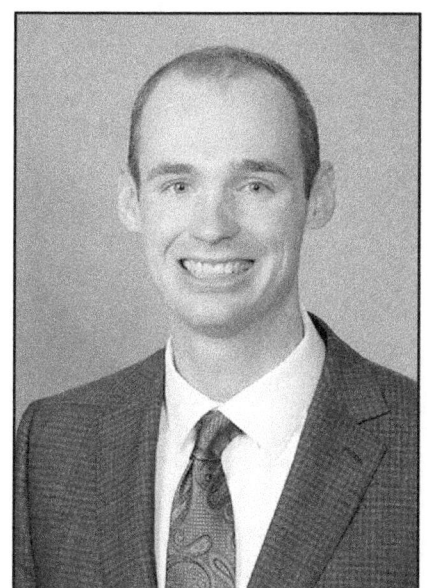

Pallavi Juneja grew up in South Brunswick, New Jersey. In 2015, she graduated from Haverford College where she played women's basketball and earned her BA in English. After two years of teaching high school English, Pallavi enrolled in Wake Forest School of Medicine. As a medical student, she began working as an editor for *in-Training*; in her fourth year, she helmed the publication as co-editor-in-chief. Pallavi graduated from medical school in May 2021 with an interest in health equity and narrative medicine. She currently lives in New York with her wife and dog and is a neurology resident at Columbia University Irving Medical Center.

Sam Rouleau is a Connecticut native. In 2017, he graduated from the U.S. Air Force Academy and subsequently matriculated to the Mayo Clinic Alix School of Medicine. As a second-year medical student, he joined the *in-Training* team and went on to serve as co-editor-in-chief during his fourth year. Sam enjoys reading and writing (mainly poetry) and sees the humanities as fundamental to the field of medicine. He is currently an emergency medicine resident at UC Davis Medical Center.

www.ingramcontent.com/pod-product-compliance
Lightning Source LLC
Chambersburg PA
CBHW031628160426
43196CB00006B/330